Alzheimer's
and Infectiou

## McFarland Health Topics

# Alzheimer's Disease and Infectious Causes

## The Theory and Evidence

ELAINE A. MOORE

MCFARLAND HEALTH TOPICS

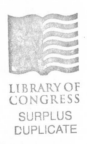

McFarland & Company, Inc., Publishers
*Jefferson, North Carolina*

This book is intended as an educational resource
and not as a substitute for medical advice.

All illustrations are by Marvin G. Miller.

ISBN (print) 978-1-4766-7861-0
ISBN (ebook) 978-1-4766-3891-1

LIBRARY OF CONGRESS AND BRITISH LIBRARY
CATALOGUING DATA ARE AVAILABLE

Library of Congress Control Number 2020005712

Front cover images © 2020 Shutterstock

Printed in the United States of America

*McFarland & Company, Inc., Publishers
Box 611, Jefferson, North Carolina 28640
www.mcfarlandpub.com*

To Rick, Lisa, Brett, Linda,
Brooklyn, and Eli—my A team

# Acknowledgments

I'm grateful to my family and friends for encouraging me to write this book and for understanding when research and writing kept me away from other activities. Special thanks are extended to Marv Miller, my dear friend and illustrator, who created all of the images in this book. My thanks are likewise extended to SammyJo Wilkinson and Randal F. Hubbard for their help in wading through an enormous amount of medical literature.

I'd also like to thank the many researchers who have worked to elucidate and explain the causes of Alzheimer's disease, especially Lawrence Broxmeyer, MD; Steven Gundry, MD; David Perlmutter, MD; Joseph Mercola, MD; Mark Hyman, MD; and Rodney Dietert, PhD. I'd also like to express my gratitude to Layla Milholen at McFarland for always being ready to answer my questions and for being patient as I deliberated for two years, waiting to find an important, fascinating, and meaningful topic to research and write about.

# Table of Contents

# Preface

When my mother was diagnosed with Alzheimer's disease (AD) in 1981, there were no effective therapies for this condition and little was known about its causes. As a clinical chemist with an interest in alternative medicine, I bought her various supplements designed to increase acetylcholine levels and improve memory. My pharmacist brother gave her medications intended to help increase cerebral blood flow. None of these therapies helped. Her gerontologist checked her thyroid, vitamin B12, and folate levels and found them to be within the normal range. All we could do was offer comfort and support as her condition deteriorated.

Over the years, I kept up with advances in AD, volunteered at a nursing home for AD patients, and wrote two books on the subject. From scrutinizing the results of studies presented at international conferences, I learned that a lack of exercise, chronic stress, and a high-sugar diet were considered contributing factors to Alzheimer's disease. These factors marginally helped to explain the probable causes in my mother's case.

However, in pondering causes, I recalled hearing about the time that my mother was paralyzed for one year when she was six years old. Too many years have passed to determine the cause of this paralysis, but I had to wonder whether my mother had suffered from reactivation of a herpes virus, particularly *Cytomegalovirus*, or if she had been infected by a variant of the polio virus or contracted *Mycobacterium avium* from the chickens our family raised. I also considered the DDT trucks that barreled through our neighborhood in the summers and the pollution from the Lake Erie fish we ate.

This past year, when my husband developed *Herpes zoster ophthalmicus* (HZO), which is a condition of shingles that affects patients' eyes, I was surprised and alarmed to find that recent studies showed a strong association with developing AD within five years. However, it was encouraging to learn that while the risk of dementia remains high, treatment with antiviral drugs reduces this risk by a factor of ten.

I was also surprised to learn that numerous viruses, bacteria, spirochetes, and fungi had been found in the brains of patients with AD. Considering that *Treponema pallidum* has long been known to cause a similar form of dementia in patients with syphilis, the pieces to this intriguing puzzle grew clearer. However, the question remained regarding whether many different microbes caused the neuroinflammation that leads to AD or if one particular organism was the true cause.

Recent research into the importance of a healthy microbiome shows that the microbes that live among us can contribute to disease when pathogenic microbes take up residence in the gut. The use of antibiotics in particular can affect the gut microbiome for years, causing a condition of dysbiosis and increasing susceptibility to viral infections and the reactivation of latent viruses. Certain genetic polymorphisms can also make these infections more likely. In addition, a number of chemicals such as non-steroidal anti-inflammatory drugs and glyphosate can injure the gut lining, causing leaky gut syndrome, which allows gut microbes to travel to the central nervous system. Permeability in the blood-brain barrier increases with age, another factor influencing the passage of microbes into the brain.

Thanks to the work of David Perlmutter, MD, we now know of the immune system changes and the alterations in the intestinal lining and blood-brain barrier that lead to neuroinflammation and dementia, and we know how to help prevent and heal these alterations with dietary interventions. In addition, thanks to advances in functional medicine, we know that there are several conditions (such as vitamin D and E deficiencies, hypothyroidism, diabetes, mitochondrial dysfunction, and vascular disorders) that can contribute to dementia and also be successfully treated.

My goal in writing this book is to introduce readers to the various microorganisms that have been implicated in the development of Alzheimer's disease along with the benefits of treatment for these conditions, including treatments that protect and nurture the microbiome. Chapters on risk factors, genes, epigenetics, nutrition, and DNA methylation are included to highlight the importance of lifestyle and environmental influences for risk reduction. It is my hope that Alzheimer's disease can ultimately be prevented and treated when its causes and contributing factors are fully addressed.

# Introduction

In 1906, Alois Alzheimer speculated that the disease affecting 51-year-old Auguste Deter, making her paranoid and suspicious, might have an infectious origin. Pressed by his director supervisor, he ignored certain findings that suggested infection and christened his patient's condition with his own name, calling it Alzheimer's disease. Alzheimer's peers shared his initial skepticism and observed that his patient had all the characteristic signs of tuberculosis. Unfortunately, without the aid of sophisticated laboratory equipment, his conjecture has remained speculation for more than one hundred years, and conditions of senile dementia have come to be known as Alzheimer's disease.

After the death of Deter at age 56, Alzheimer studied her brain and identified the hallmark brain changes that characterize Alzheimer's disease (AD): the amyloid beta plaques and neurofibrillary tau protein tangles. Other researchers—notably Oskar Fischer, Alzheimer's main rival—observed the presence of bacteria and commented that amyloid plaque deposits are seen in the brains of patients with infections. Later studies showed that Deter had none of the genetic markers for Alzheimer's disease.

In the 1980s, infection was again considered as the causative agent in AD. However, with the identification of amyloid beta plaque and its derivation from amyloid precursor protein (APP), therapies for AD have focused on reducing, blocking or eliminating these amyloid plaque deposits. To date, these therapies have ultimately met with virtually no success. This result has prompted researchers to realize that an underlying cause responsible for the neuronal changes needed to be identified.

In recent years, through studying frozen brain tissue from Alzheimer's disease patients stored in "brain banks," researchers have found that these specimens commonly contain microbes, particularly viruses, bacteria, fungi and protozoa. To a lesser extent, some microorganisms have also been found in the brains of age-matched control subjects. It appears that reactivation of viruses and persistent infection with bacteria, fungi, and protozoa can initiate a chronic immune system response that leads to an inflammatory process in the brain known as neuroinflammation, which results in neurodegenerative changes. In addition, genome-wide association studies show that this neuroinflammation is the driving force rather than a consequence of the disease process in AD.

Technological advances have also provided greater insight into the role that the immune system (particularly its response to infections) plays in AD development. Immune system changes such as increased microglial brain cell activation and activation of complement seen in patients with AD are consistent with changes seen in infection. These advances have also shown that the human body is inhabited by trillions of bacteria and other microbes that are necessary for life. Typically confined to the gut, skin, nose, mouth, and vagina, they digest food; produce hormones, essential vitamins, and neurotransmitters; and help eliminate waste. However, when conditions of leaky gut syndrome, defects in the blood-brain barrier, or mitochondrial dysfunction occur, these organisms easily make their way into the brain, setting the stage for neurodegeneration.

Amyloid beta protein has recently been found to be an antimicrobial agent that the body produces in response to infection as an early step in the immune response. Amyloid beta protein offers early benefits in fighting infection, but subsequently, when the infection spirals out of control, this protein directly leads to the production of the destructive amyloid beta oligomers, neuroinflammation and neuronal destruction.

Amyloid beta oligomers have been found to be more toxic to neurons and their synaptic connections than the dreaded senile plaque deposits. To the surprise of researchers, many amyloid plaque deposits have also been found in the postmortem brains of elderly individuals with no symptoms of dementia. Researchers have likewise discovered that the specific pathway that the amyloid precursor protein (the progenitor of amyloid beta protein) takes directly influences whether the toxic form of amyloid beta protein is produced and senile plaques are formed.

While most studies have focused on herpes viruses as causative agents, many other viruses, bacteria, spirochetes, protozoa and fungi have also been implicated. While senile dementia has previously been known to occur in cases of syphilis and meningitis, the ability to study the brain in greater detail has led to the discovery that microorganisms—particularly herpes viruses and bacteria found in the oral cavity—are very common in the brains of individuals with AD and are also present in individuals with normal cognitive function.

*Mycobacterium* species are difficult to detect without specific laboratory tests that are ordered if *Mycobacterium* is suspected. These microbes are not detected in a routine culture and sensitivity test. With more than 190 *Mycobacterium* species in existence, and *Mycobacterium tuberculosis* the world's most prevalent infection, along with the fact that a persistent infection can linger for years without apparent symptoms, the role of *Mycobacterium* in association with secondary infectious organisms needs to be considered, and its association with AD is described in this book.

This book serves as an introduction to the microbes that live among us, the genes associated with Alzheimer's disease, the communication system between the gut and the brain, and the role of the immune system in launching an inflammatory response against infection, which can ultimately lead to AD.

Included is a description of the changes in the microbiome seen in individuals with AD, the ways in which leaky gut syndrome can lead to infection and damage the blood-brain barrier, and the association with immune system components such as decreased complement levels and reduced plasmalogen levels that are seen in AD. The primary focus is the relevance of the studies that support the infectious disease theory of AD. This book also describes supporting evidence from research studies, the results of genetic studies, and information regarding risk factors, and it includes a chapter on holistic healing and AD prevention.

While less than 1 percent of the cases of Alzheimer's disease are directly caused by genes, the other cases can be associated with environmental causes such as high blood glucose levels, vascular disease, heavy metal toxicity, damage to the blood-brain barrier, mitochondrial dysfunction, lack of exercise, nutrient deficiencies, environmental toxins, and stress. The increased susceptibility to environmental assault seen in individuals with predisposing genes for late-onset AD is also described. Studies likewise suggest that through treatment for the causative microorganism, the development and progression of Alzheimer's disease can be halted.

This book is not intended as a substitute for a proper diagnosis and treatment of AD. Rather, it is intended to help educate and empower individuals in need of more information regarding Alzheimer's disease and related conditions of dementia.

# ONE

# The Mystery of the Mind and Consciousness

Since ancient times physicians and philosophers have struggled to understand what exactly constitutes the mind as well as the conscious state. As for an understanding of consciousness, this question has been thoroughly explored, yet remains unanswered. Regarding the intricacies behind what constitutes the mind and thought processing and memory, these mysteries are described in this chapter along with a description of the normal brain as well as the neural and physical changes that characterize the brain in Alzheimer's disease (AD).

While these changes have been apparent for more than one hundred years, the causes of Alzheimer's disease, which were recognized many years ago but overlooked, have now come to light. Considering that little was known about the mysteries of the mind until the 1990s, it's not surprising that the causes of AD have remained elusive.

As Eric R. Kandel and colleagues write in *The Principles of Neural Science*, the dominant brain hemisphere sometimes interferes with the function of the other hemisphere, making it difficult to determine which mental functions are controlled by which specific function of the brain. Only since the mid–1990s have researchers had the proper tools to determine how specific mental activities are represented (Kandel et al. 2000, 16).

Very little was known about the brain prior to the 18th century. In ancient Egypt, for instance, physicians thought that the seat of intelligence resided within the heart. For this reason, during the mummification process physicians would remove the brain but leave the heart inside the body. In ancient Greece, Aristotle proposed that the brain functioned to cool the blood.

The philosopher René Descartes (1596–1650) regarded the relationship of the brain to the body as that of a machine, comparing the brain to an organ in a church. As a result of this theory, he became the founder of mind-body dualism, a school of thought christened by the philosopher's Latinized name:

Cartesianism. But while Descartes became famous for stating, "I think, therefore I am," in the late 20th century philosophers such as John Searle, whose findings took on a more scientific approach, realized that Descartes had it backward. The correct view is "I am, therefore I think" (Kandel 2018, 4). By this time, the brain's functional units—neurons—had been identified, and researchers had learned that neurons in different parts of the brain had different functions and were able to communicate with one another to produce thoughts.

## Neurons

Before the invention of the compound microscope in the 18th century, nervous tissue (tissue of the central nervous system, including the brain and spinal cord) was thought to function in the same manner as a gland. With the aid of the microscope, it became clear that nervous tissue consisted of a network of cell bodies (neurons), with axons on one end and dendrites on the other, and that the cells communicated with one another through signals sent to connections known as synapses. In the late 1700s, the Italian physician, biologist, and philosopher Luigi Galvani discovered that intact living muscle and nerve cells have the ability to produce electricity. The activity of one neuron was found to affect adjacent neurons in predictable ways. In 1780, Galvani discovered that the muscles of dead frogs' legs twitched when struck by an electrical spark, an experiment still repeated in college biology courses.

In the early 19th century, Jacob Meleschott stated that the brain produces what is known as the mind. With the idea that the brain was involved in thought, the elusive search for how thoughts are produced continued, focusing on the mysteries of the brain and the thought process. Around this time, researchers discovered that drugs do not react with cells directly. Instead, drugs and other chemicals (including the body's messenger chemicals known as neurotransmitters, such as serotonin) react with protein receptors.

Receptors are usually found on the surface membrane of cells; occasionally they are found on the cell nucleus. Like a key fitting a lock, a chemical that binds to the receptor is given entry into the cell, where it can carry out its intended actions. Specific compounds can only react with certain receptors. This finding suggested a chemical basis as well as an electrical basis for communication between the cells of the central nervous system. With advances in diagnostic imaging tests, it is now known that communication between interconnected cells is responsible for behavioral responses.

In 1928, Edgar Adrian (a pioneer in the electrophysiological study of the nervous system and a recipient of the 1932 Nobel Prize in Physiology or Medicine) surgically exposed a small nerve with attached axons from the neck of an anesthetized rabbit. He removed most of the axons and placed an electrode on the remaining ones. Every time the rabbit took a breath, Adrian noticed a flurry of electrical activity. By attaching a loudspeaker, he was able to hear clicking noises that turned out to be an electrical signal known as an action potential as neurons communicated. From this result, Adrian deduced that the inside of the membrane that surrounds a neuron and its axis contains a slightly negative charge relative to the outside. Because of the unequal distribution of ions, each neuron is able to function as a tiny battery, storing electricity to be used as needed (Kandel 2018, 17).

## The Thought Process

Today it's known that electrical activity, along with the release of chemical neurotransmitters (such as acetylcholine), combined with changes in specific cellular contacts and alterations in neuronal activity, lead to the process of thought. According to the Neuron Doctrine, each neuron is a unique element and serves as the fundamental building block and signaling unit of the brain. Neurons only interact with other neurons at synapses, forming intricate networks known as neural circuits, allowing communication from one cell to another only at particular sites. Because of this connection specificity, the brain has a precise circuitry that underlies complex tasks such as perception, action, and thought. Most important, information flows in one direction only, from the dendrites to the cell body to the axon, and then along the axon to the synapse. This flow of information is known as dynamic polarization (Kandel 2018, 16–17).

Brain scans enable researchers to see which specific areas of the brain light up when individuals think, are stimulated, solve math equations or listen to music. With a functional scanner, patients with chronic pain can be coached to control activity in the front of their brains in an effort to reduce pain. It's also known that there are 1,000 × 1,000 billion points at which neurons connect with one another at junctions known as synapses. These connections occur through over 60,000 miles of nerve fiber (Swaab 2014, 6).

## *Neuroscience*

Neuroscience—the study of the structure and function of the cells that make up the central nervous system—is a relatively new discipline that first came into use in the 1960s by scientific visionaries, key among them the Massachusetts Institute of Technology neurophysiologist Francis Schmidt. Encompassing various disciplines, including cellular and molecular biology, anatomy, physiology, biochemistry genetics, informatics and psychology, neuroscientists seek to understand the brain's relationship to the rest of the mind and body and present a unified way of studying the central nervous system. Prior to the 21st century, physicians who specialized in studying the brain were known as neuroanatomists and neurophysiologists. In studying the structure and function of the brain's components, early specialists developed various theories as to the relationship between the brain and behavior.

Early researchers led the way until eventually the specific functions of certain areas of the brain were matched and mapped. The French physician Pierre Paul Broca (1824–1880) specialized in patients with brain damage. He was the first to recognize that different regions of the brain controlled specific functions. He discovered that damage to the forward part of the left hemisphere allowed those so afflicted to understand language although they could no longer express themselves, instead communicating with indistinguishable mumbles. Today the part of the brain that controls speech is known as Broca's area. Similarly, Broca's colleague, Carl Wernicke, discovered that damage in the rear part of the left hemisphere (now called Wernicke's area) caused those affected to no longer comprehend language, although they could speak freely, if not logically. Although the brain circuitry for language was eventually found to be even more complex than Broca and Wernicke realized, their early findings formed the basis of our modern view of the neurology of language and neurological disorders.

In 1873, Camillo Golgi in Italy developed a stain using silver chromate salt to help examine neurons (nervous system cells) microscopically. In 1898, Golgi discovered cell organelles, which he named Golgi bodies, and discovered that these microscopic structures convert carbohydrates and lipids into cellular energy. In the early 20th century, Santiago Ramón y Cajal, a Spanish pathologist, discovered that neurons are independent functioning units that constitute a large interconnected network. In 1906, Golgi and Cajal jointly received the Nobel Prize in Physiology or Medicine for their work categorizing neurons in the brain.

## Papal Conference on the Brain and Conscious Experience

By 1964, the intricacies of the brain still remained a mystery. For this reason, from September 28 through October 4, 1964, the Pontifical Academy in Rome hosted a weeklong workshop on the topic of "Brain and Conscious Experience." The idea was to gather the world's top researchers to present their findings and theories on what constituted consciousness in a way that would link the field of psychology to what would come to be the neurosciences. The renowned physician and physiologist Sir John Eccles from Australia was chosen to lead the workshop.

In 1925, Eccles had studied at Oxford with the famed neurophysiologist Charles Sherrington, whose work on neurons earned him the 1932 Nobel Prize in Physiology or Medicine. Sherrington coined the term *synapse* to describe the gap between neurons, and he was a powerful influence on Eccles's future work. After receiving his PhD in 1929, Eccles went on to study the method of neural transmission at the synapses. Initially, Eccles presumed that all cellular transmission was electrical. However, through rigorous testing of his hypothesis, he determined that synaptic transmission was in fact chemical.

Over the next decade, Eccles went on to elucidate the mechanisms involved in the firing and inhibiting of motor neuron synapses in the spinal cord. From there, he began to study the cells of the thalamus, hippocampus and cerebellum. In 1958, he was appointed a knight bachelor for his research. In 1963, for his work on motor neuron synapses, he was awarded the Nobel Prize in Physiology or Medicine.

A natural choice to head the papal conference, Eccles was able to select a team of medical experts with the stipulation that the team would not include philosophers. Prior to the meeting, the participants were given a brief by the Papal Academy. In this brief, consciousness was described as "the psycho-physiological concept of perpetual capacity, of awareness of perception and the ability to act and react accordingly" (Ganziga 2018, 66).

During the conference, while discussing cerebral events as related to conscious experience, Eccles asked how some specific spatiotemporal pattern of neuronal activity in the cerebral cortex evoked a particular sensory experience. The answer still remains unknown. At the end of the conference week, a summation was given to MIT psychologist Hans-Lukes Teuber, one of the founding fathers of neuropsychology. While the conference hadn't solved the mind-body problem, in 1966 Eccles published the papal conference's findings in his landmark book, *Brain and Conscious Experience*. While the scientists were able to easily explain the process of perception, the matter in which thoughts became memories was a subject of debate. The possible role of synaptic factors in producing memory was discussed, but without the sophisticated imaging tests available today, definitive proof remained elusive (Eccles 1966, 549).

In 1966, Eccles moved to the United States and worked as a professor at the University of Buffalo before retiring and moving to Switzerland, where he died at the age of 94 in 1997. In 1991, Eccles wrote his master achievement, *Evolution of the Brain, Creation of the Self*, which describes the Darwinian evolution of the human brain and mind over time, particularly in relation to the brain's motor and linguistic skills.

With the 1973 discovery of the opiate receptor by Candace Pert, the brain's response to chemical neurotransmitters as well as drugs provided the information Eccles had been searching for. He writes that while genes determine the makeup of the brain, it is life's experiences and influences that make each individual, as well as their thoughts and memories, unique (Eccles 1991, 237). This finding is especially pertinent in connection with Alzheimer's disease, in which a variety of genes are associated with late-onset Alzheimer's disease (LOAD), although having them does not mean that an individual will develop AD. Alois Alzheimer's first patient, Auguste Deter, who developed AD in her early fifties after experiencing significant weight loss and delusions, had none of the genes now known to be associated with LOAD or early-onset AD (EOAD), which is defined as AD occurring before the age of 65 years.

The normal functioning of the central nervous system is introduced in the following sections to demonstrate the processes that lead to behavior and thought processes. This discussion is followed by a description of the cellular changes that occur in the brain affected by AD. These changes, which interfere with normal neuronal signaling, ultimately result in the mental and behavioral symptoms that characterize AD.

## The Central Nervous System

The central nervous system serves as the body's command center for mediating behavior. The central nervous system consists of the brain and the spinal cord. With consideration for the brain's major components, the central nervous system is reported to have seven major divisions: the spinal cord, the brain's medulla, pons, cerebellum, midbrain, diencephalon and cerebral hemispheres (or telencephalon).

The brain's major components are found in both hemispheres of the brain, although they may differ in size and shape. The neurons in different parts of the central nervous system are similar, but the number and types of neurons and the ways in which they are interconnected differ. Behavior results from the pattern in which appropriately connected cells signal (and thereby communicate with) one another. Neurons in different parts of the brain have specialized functions that they carry out upon receiving signals from other parts of the brain. As the command center, sensory neurons in the brain receive stimuli from the environment, process this information, and communicate it throughout the body.

For instance, in driving a car, visual information that we take in while watching oncoming traffic combines with sensory information from our body, such as the way we're sitting or how relaxed we are. This information

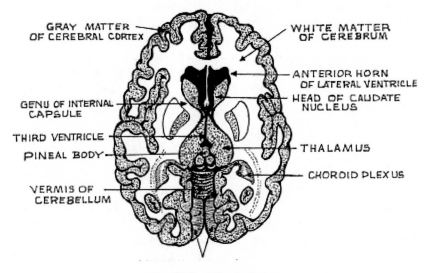

GRAY MATTER OF CEREBRAL CORTEX

WHITE MATTER OF CEREBRUM

ANTERIOR HORN OF LATERAL VENTRICLE

GENU OF INTERNAL CAPSULE

HEAD OF CAUDATE NUCLEUS

THIRD VENTRICLE

PINEAL BODY

THALAMUS

CHOROID PLEXUS

VERMIS OF CEREBELLUM

**Cerebellar Hemispheres.**

is sent to a multisensory processing region in the central cortex and synchronized with earlier memories (of past driving and related experiences) to guide us in choosing the best behavioral response.

This information is combined with previous information stored in the amygdala, a structure located in the temporal lobe primarily concerned with memory, emotions, survival instincts and social behavior. Neurons in the amygdala participate in the processing response and activate the autonomous nervous system to prepare the body for action. This program then reverts to the primary motor cortex, where commands from the brain reach motor neurons located in the muscles of the arms, back, shoulders, legs and hands. Thus, in a finely synchronized orchestration between multiple interconnected neurons, the body is able to react properly without dwelling over each step in the behavioral process.

The peripheral nervous system, while intertwined with the central nervous system, is a separate entity consisting of the nerves and ganglia located outside of the central nervous system. Information supplied by the environment (both the external environment and the internal environment of the body) is transmitted from the peripheral nervous system to the central nervous system.

The peripheral nervous system is subdivided into somatic and autonomic divisions. The somatic division includes the sensory neurons that innervate the skin, muscles and joints. The cell bodies of these sensory neurons are located in the dorsal root ganglia and the cranial ganglia. The autonomic division mediates both visceral sensation and motor control of the viscera, smooth muscles, and exocrine glands. It comprises the sympathetic, para-sympathetic, and enteric systems. The sympathetic system is known for participating in the body's reaction to stress, while the parasympathetic system works to conserve body resources and maintain homeostasis. The enteric nervous system manages the smooth muscle contractions of the gut during digestion and communicates with neurons in the central and peripheral nervous systems.

## The Brain

The brain in its entirety weighs about three pounds and is composed of about 100 billion neurons and 10–50 times as many glial (immune system) cells. Glial cells, which play an important role in inflammation, were once thought to be glue-like, serving to hold neurons together. Now it's known that glial cells are immune system cells that help protect neurons. In addition, they are crucial to the transfer of chemical messages and consequently to all brain processes, including the formation of long-term memories. Albert Einstein was known to have an unusually large number of glial cells (Swaab 2014, 4). The brain uses about 20 percent of the body's energy reserves.

## The Spinal Cord

The spinal cord extends from the base of the skull to the first lumbar vertebra situated in the lower back. The spinal cord contains motor neurons responsible for voluntary and reflex movements and is able to process information sent from the skin, joints, back and muscles of the trunk and limbs. The spinal cord varies in size and shape depending on whether its motor neurons extend to the limbs or to the trunk. The spinal cord and the brain are surrounded by and bathed in a clear, colorless liquid called spinal fluid. Spinal fluid is produced by a group of cells called the choroid plexus, which resides deep inside the brain. In Alzheimer's disease and other neurological disorders, changes in the chemical composition of spinal fluid can be measured and used as aids in disease diagnosis.

## The Brain Stem

The medulla, pons, and midbrain are collectively referred to as the brain stem. The brain stem lies continuous with the spinal cord and contains distinct clusters of neurons needed for various motor and sensory systems. Signals from the brain stem can be sent and received from ascending and descending pathways. The brain stem is primarily concerned with sensations arising from the head, neck and face and the associated motor control of these structures.

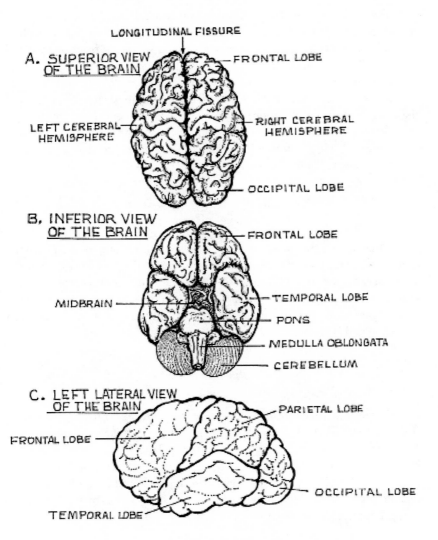

**The Adult Brain.**

The brain stem is also the point of entry for specialized signals associated with hearing, balance, and taste. Motor neurons found in the brain stem control many parasympathetic or autonomous functions, such as cardiac output, blood pressure, peristalsis of the gut, and constriction of the pupils.

The medulla is situated near the top of the spinal cord and shares many of its functions. Clusters of neurons in the medulla assist in regulating blood pressure and respiration. Other neuronal groups are involved in taste, hearing and balance as well as the control of neck and facial muscles.

The pons lies above the medulla and protrudes from the underlying surface of the brain stem. Clusters of neurons called pontine nuclei are involved with relaying information about movement and sensation from the cerebral cortex to the cerebellum. Clusters of neurons on the upper side of the pons are involved in respiration, taste and sleep.

The smallest part of the brain stem, the midbrain, is situated in front of the pons. Neurons in the midbrain connect to components of the motor systems, particularly those in the cerebellum, the basal ganglia, and the cerebral hemispheres. The substantia nigra, which represents the nucleus of the midbrain, provides input to a portion of the basal ganglia that regulates voluntary movements.

## Cerebellum

Situated over the pons, the cerebellum contains more neurons than the other subdivisions of the brain, including the cerebral hemispheres. However, since there few neuronal types present in the cerebellum, its connections are well understood. Its primary roles are maintaining posture and receiving input regarding balance from neurons in the inner ears. It is also involved in cognition and language skills.

## Diencephalon

The diencephalon has two major components: the thalamus and the hypothalamus. The thalamus helps integrate information regarding movement from the cerebellum and basal ganglia and transmits this information to the cerebral hemispheres. The hypothalamus regulates behaviors essential for homeostasis (bodily systems working together to maintain health) and reproduction. The hypothalamus exerts control over several bodily functions, including growth, eating, drinking and maternal behavior, by regulating the hormones secreted by the pituitary gland.

## Cerebral Hemispheres

The right and left cerebral hemispheres represent the largest region of the brain. The hemispheres house the cerebral cortex, white matter, and three underlying structures: the basal ganglia, the amygdala, and the hippocampal formation. The hemispheres regulate perception, motor, and cognitive functions, including memory and emotion. The hemispheres are connected by the corpus callosum, a network of fibers that connect symmetrical regions in both hemispheres. The cerebral hemispheres each have four lobes: the frontal, parietal, temporal and occipital lobes.

The cerebral cortex, which is also known as the cerebrum, is a thin outer layer surrounding the cerebral hemispheres. It is composed of folded gray matter and plays an important role in consciousness. It is responsible for most of the planning and execution of daily actions. As the most highly developed part of the brain, it is responsible for thinking, perceiving, and producing language. The cerebral cortex has a highly convoluted shape formed by grooves known as sulci that separate the elevated regions known as gyri.

## The Entorhinal Cortex

While there are many subdivisions in the lobes of the cerebral hemispheres, an introduction to the entorhinal cortex is important because it is the area in which the earliest changes due to AD first appear. The entorhinal cortex is located in the medial temporal lobe and functions as a central hub in a widespread neuronal network connected to the hippocampus; it is involved in the creation of memory, navigation and the perception of time.

## Neurons and Glial Cells

Besides neurons, the tissues of the central nervous system are composed of 10–50 times as many immune system cells collectively referred to as glial cells. Glial cells include astrocytes and microglial cells. In AD, cells of the nervous system, primarily the neurons along with their synapses, are damaged and destroyed. In addition, injury to glial cells prevents them from carrying out their protective functions.

The cellular components of the brain and the interconnections between its cells are established during embryonic and postnatal development. The development of the nervous system also depends on the expression of particular genes at particular places and times during development. The factors that control the differentiation of neurons arise both from cellular sources within the embryo and from the external environment. The diverse functions of the nervous system, ranging from sensory perception to motivation and memory, depend on precise connections formed between distinct types of nerve cells. Once they are recruited, cells from the ectoderm's neural plate of progenitor cells begin to acquire differentiated properties that lead to their development as either neurons or glial cells.

The human brain contains about 100 billion neurons and ten times as many glial cells. Among the neurons, there are reported to be hundreds of different neuronal types, with more differentiation seen in the brain than in other organs of the body. This differentiation occurs as cells from the ectoderm form a neural plate, a column of epithelial cells. These embryological

MACROGLIA

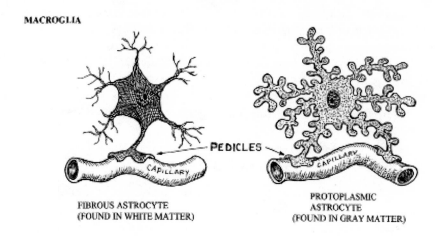

FIBROUS ASTROCYTE
(FOUND IN WHITE MATTER)

PROTOPLASMIC
ASTROCYTE
(FOUND IN GRAY MATTER)

MICROGLIA

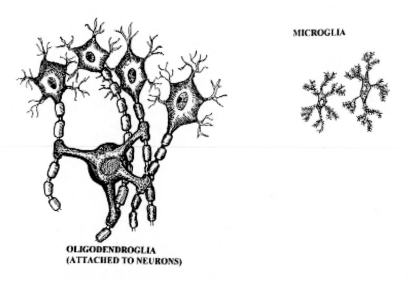

OLIGODENDROGLIA
(ATTACHED TO NEURONS)

**Astrocytes and Microglial Cells.**

cells then align and form a neural tube. Cells not recruited for the nervous system become skin cells. Depending on their placement along the neural tube, cells are recruited for the forebrain, midbrain, or hindbrain. Signaling molecules from other central nervous system cells influence the differentiation of new cells.

Neurons, which are found in the central nervous system and nerve ganglia (as well as the enteric nervous system in the gastrointestinal tract), contain cell bodies or soma with extensions (axons and dendrites). Varying in size from 4 to 100 microns, neurons have a length ranging from several millimeters to several feet. Neurons are capable of transmitting nerve signals to and from the brain at a rate of 200 miles per hour. The neuronal cell body contains cytoplasm surrounding a centrally located large cell nucleus. A compound called Nissl substance found in the cytoplasm is responsible for producing protein and distributing it to the axons and dendrites. Many types of neurons with specific functions exist, and different types are generally grouped together by location.

Each neuron has one axon and about 100,000 dendrites. Neurons send out axons and dendrites in all directions throughout their network and communicate with other axons and dendrites located on cells in other locations. These cellular connections intertwine, but do not touch, to form an interconnected tangle with 100 trillion constantly changing connections. Neurons in

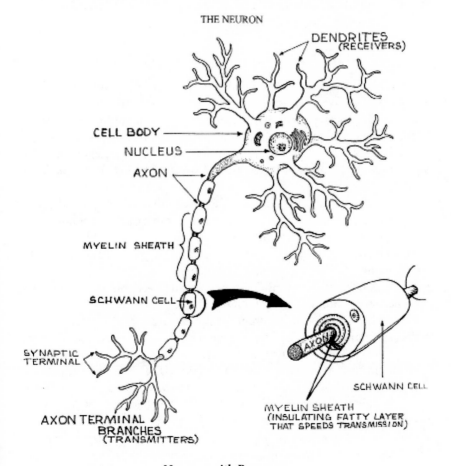

THE NEURON

**Neurons with Processes.**

specific areas of the brain become dysfunctional or injured in AD, leading to a disruption in these connections and a corresponding loss of their intended functions.

GLIAL CELLS

Glial cells (glia) are immune system cells that make up approximately 90 percent of the cells found within the brain. The ratio of glial cells to neurons varies widely, although glial cells always outnumber neurons and there are typically 50 times more glial cells than neurons in the central nervous system. Several subtypes of glial cells exist, each with distinct functions, including astrocytes, oligodendrocytes, ependymal cells, Schwann cells, microglia, and satellite cells. Glial cells primarily function to surround neurons and hold them in place, to supply nutrients and oxygen to neurons, to insulate neurons from one another, and to defend against, destroy, engulf, and remove the carcasses of dead neurons.

## The Neurotransmitter Acetylcholine

Neurotransmitters include a family of chemicals involved in the signals sent between neurons. These signals are necessary for thought and learning processes. The message sent to a cell (the postsynaptic cell) doesn't depend on the chemical nature of the transmitter; rather, it depends on the specific cell receptor that receives the chemical message. Acetylcholine, which is produced by cholinergic neurons, was the first neurotransmitter to be discovered.

Acetylcholine has the ability to excite some postsynaptic cells and inhibit others. In some other cells, acetylcholine can both excite and inhibit. This neurotransmitter is found at the neuromuscular junction (which connects nerve cells to muscles cells) in autonomic ganglia and at parasympathetic nerve endings. In the neuromuscular junction, acetylcholine is released at the endings of motor neurons. With inadequate acetylcholine, the nervous system cannot communicate with muscle cells.

Acetylcholine also helps brain cells communicate with each other by facilitating communication from the basal forebrain to the cerebral cortex and hippocampus, aiding the learning and memory processes. In addition, acetylcholine regulates sleeps and facilitates higher cognitive functions. Acetylcholine deficiency can predispose an individual to a number of different neurological disorders, including AD. The effect of acetylcholine is limited by the enzyme acetylcholinesterase and by the number of cell receptors that are able to bind with acetylcholine. Normally, acetylcholinesterase destroys any remaining acetylcholine after its initial use, preventing its reuptake.

THE ACTION OF THE NEUROTRANSMITTER ACETYLCHOLINE

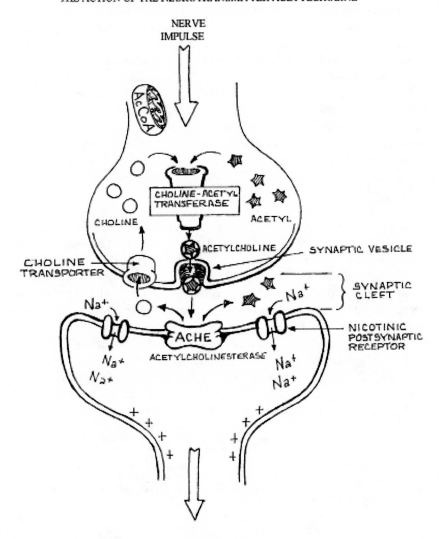

**Acetylcholine.**

## The Brain in Alzheimer's Disease

AD is the most common form of dementia. Other causes/forms of dementia include cerebrovascular disease, frontotemporal dementia (FTD), multi-infarct dementia, Lewy body dementia, Parkinson's disease, Creutzfeldt-Jakob disease, mixed dementia, Hashimoto's encephalopathy, posterior cortical atrophy, vitamin B1 (thiamine) deficiency in Wernicke-Korsakoff syndrome in alcoholism, brain tumors, vitamin B12 deficiency, infections such as AIDS and encephalitis, and normal pressure hydrocephalus. The only way to confirm AD is with postmortem brain studies, although certain imaging and laboratory tests can be performed to help support a probable AD diagnosis. With sophisticated testing, AD is now confirmed with postmortem studies in more than 90 percent of cases (Kandel et al. 2000, 1152).

The primary changes found in the brains of patients with AD are also present in the brains of elderly dementia-free brains, although in dementia-free patients these changes usually occur to a significantly lesser degree and at more advanced ages. However, in many cases the number of senile plaques in the normal brain is the same as that found in patients with AD. In several respects, AD can be viewed as a premature, accelerated and severe process of brain aging (Swaab 2014, 340).

In addition, it's known that some weakening of memory, beginning at around age forty, is normal and expected. This memory loss, which is called benign senescent forgetfulness or age-related memory loss, is similar to that seen in the early stages of Alzheimer's disease (mild cognitive impairment). Eric Kandel and his colleagues at Columbia University conducted studies with mice to see what aspects of this memory loss differed. Although mice do not develop Alzheimer's disease, they show an age-related memory loss that is centered in the hippocampus. The researchers discovered that while symptoms are similar, age-related memory loss is related to changes occurring in the brain's dentate nucleus in a gene called RbA48 (Kandel 2018, 116).

In addition, a Columbia University geneticist, Gerard Karsenty, found that bone is an endocrine organ that releases a hormone called osteocalcin. Osteocalcin acts on many organs, including the brain, where it promotes

Brain Cells in Alzheimer's Disease.

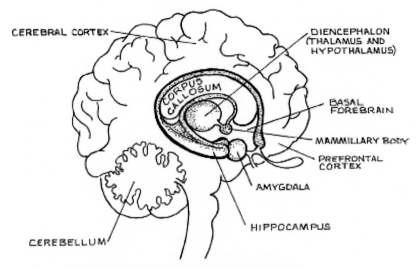

CEREBRAL CORTEX

DIENCEPHALON
(THALAMUS AND
HYPOTHALAMUS)

CORPUS CALLOSUM

BASAL FOREBRAIN

MAMMILLARY BODY

PREFRONTAL CORTEX

AMYGDALA

HIPPOCAMPUS

CEREBELLUM

☆ THE CEREBRAL CORTEX IS INVOLVED IN CONSCIOUS
THOUGHT AND LANGUAGE

☆ THE BASAL FOREBRAIN IS IMPORTANT IN MEMORY
AND LEARNING, AND CONSISTS OF NUMEROUS
NEURONS CONTAINING ACETYLCHOLINE.

☆ THE HIPPOCAMPUS IS ESSENTIAL TO MEMORY STORAGE

The Memory Center.

spatial memory and learning by influencing the production of various neurotransmitters as well as proteins needed for memory formation. Exercise is known to increase osteocalcin production, which may be the reason why exercise benefits the human brain.

As part of the experiment on normal aging versus AD, mice were treated with osteocalcin. The treated mice showed definite improvement in memory tasks. Also, young mice treated with osteocalcin showed improved learning capabilities when compared to untreated mice. These studies show that age-related memory loss is distinct from AD and acts on different processes in a separate region of the brain. Kandel writes, "Wisdom and perspective certainly increase with age. Anxiety tends to decrease. The challenge for all of us is to maximize the benefits of aging while doing our best to minimize the downside" (Kandel 2018, 117).

## Characteristic Brain Changes in AD

In 1906, Alois Alzheimer noted specific brain changes in the first patient with AD. This patient was a 51-year-old woman who had developed memory deficits along with a progressive loss of her cognitive abilities. Unable to orient herself in her own home, she was institutionalized for five years before dying. These changes included atrophy of the cerebral cortices, extracellular (outside the cell wall) deposits of senile amyloid beta (Aβ) plaque, and intracellular (within the cells) neurofibrillary tangles (NFTs) in the cells of the neocortex and hippocampus.

Understanding the complex brain changes that occur in AD is important for understanding the various therapies that target these changes. Abnormal brain changes in AD selectively affect neurons in specific regions of the brain, primarily the neocortex, the entorhinal area, hippocampus, amygdala, nucleus basalis, anterior thalamus, and several brain stem monoaminergic nuclei, such as the locus ceruleus and raphe complex (Kandel et al. 2000, 1152).

The main characteristics seen in AD include gross cortical atrophy, ventricular dilatation, the presence of amyloid beta protein in senile plaque deposits, and intraneuronal tangles of hyperphosphorylated tau protein (neurofibrillary tangles). In areas of the brain that are damaged, the dysfunction and death of neurons result in a reduction of synaptic proteins, preventing cells from communicating with one another. Ultimately the cholinergic neurons in the nucleus basalis, medial septal nucleus, and diagonal band of Broca, which provide the main cholinergic pathways to the neocortex and hippocampus, are destroyed. For this reason, early treatments focused on increasing acetylcholinesterase (also called cholinesterase) levels.

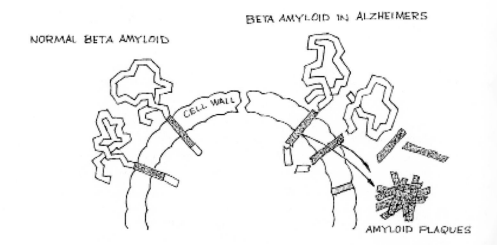

**Plaque Formation.**

## Acetylcholine Deficiency and Cholinesterase Inhibitors

In the early stages of AD, a select group of cholinergic neurons in the cortex and hippocampus become deficient in the neurotransmitter acetylcholine. Acetylcholine is one of the body's main neurotransmitters and sends signals to both the central and the peripheral nervous systems. Among acetylcholine's numerous functions, it transmits chemical signals that cause muscles to contract, activates signals that cause the sensation of pain, helps to regulate various endocrine functions and regulates the rapid eye movement (REM) phase of sleep. Because acetylcholine transmits signals involved in learning, memory and attention, acetylcholine deficiency is thought to interfere with the processes of learning and memory in AD patients.

After acetylcholine transmits its intended signals, excess acetylcholine remains at the postsynaptic terminal. Normally, the enzyme acetylcholinesterase (more commonly referred to as cholinesterase) breaks down acetylcholine very rapidly to prevent postsynaptic nerves from being excessively stimulated. Drugs that prevent acetylcholine from being broken down are called cholinesterase blockers or cholinesterase inhibitors and effectively increase both the amount and the duration of action of acetylcholine. Cholinesterase inhibitors were one of the earliest treatments for AD. The drugs tacrine (Cognex), galantamine (Razadyne ER, Reminyl), and donepezil (Aricept) are examples of cholinesterase inhibitors.

## Neurofibrillary Tangles

In affected nerve cells, the cytoskeleton is frequently altered primarily by the presence of neurofibrillary tangles (NFTs). These are inclusions of twisted fibers that occur in the cell bodies and proximal dendrites that contain paired helical filaments and 15-nanometer straight filaments. Composed of poorly soluble hyperphosphorylated isoforms of tau, a microtubule-binding protein that is normally soluble, NFTs interfere with the ability of neurons to communicate with other cells. Because the cytoskeleton is essential for maintaining cellular structure and the intracellular transfer of proteins and organelles, including transport along axons, NFTs compromise the functions of synaptic inputs and the viability of neurons. The inability of neurons to communicate leads to deficits in thought processing and memory.

Theories suggesting that AD results from the widespread presence of NFTs are proposed by scientists called tauists because of the abnormalities seen in tau protein in patients with AD. However, NFTs are also seen in other conditions of dementia, which are known as tauopathies. Besides AD, other tauopathies include progressive supranuclear palsy (PSP), frontotemporal lobar degeneration (FLTD-TAU), and corticobasal degeneration. A restricted presence of NFTs in neurons that produce dopamine is likewise present in Parkinson's disease. In smaller numbers, NFTs are also present in elderly individuals as a result of the aging process.

## Amyloid Beta Protein (Aβ)

Amyloid beta protein—which is also known as Aβ (the term used here)—β-amyloid, and beta amyloid protein are generic names for a class of sticky proteins found in the extracellular plaque deposits brains of individuals with AD and other conditions. Aβ consists of 38–43 amino acids, and the number of amino acids present is under the control of several different genes.

The longer forms of Aβ, particularly those that end in 42 amino acids, have an increased propensity to aggregate into polymers and plaque deposits that produce neuronal damage. Aβ is produced by all of the body's cells during normal cell metabolism and is not unique to neurons. Blood levels of Aβ primarily occur from smooth muscle. Recent studies show that Aβ has antimicrobial properties, which are described in Chapter Two, and is produced during normal cell metabolism. Its production is increased in response to infections and trauma.

Deposits of Aβ are found in the brains of normal elderly subjects, although they are generally less widespread than the deposits seen in individuals with AD and other neurodegenerative disorders. Aggregates of Aβ characterize many, if not all, neurodegenerative disorders, not just AD and Parkinson's disease but also the prion disorder Creutzfeldt-Jakob disease; various motor neuron diseases such as amyotrophic lateral sclerosis; the large group of polyglutamine disorders, including Huntington's disease; and diseases of peripheral tissue such as familial amyloid polyneuropathy (FAP).

Aβ is derived from another protein, known as amyloid precursor protein (APP). The path that APP takes to form the subtypes of Aβ is influenced by various factors, including infection. This process is described in Chapter Two along with the infection hypothesis of AD. The notion that AD is directly caused by increased Aβ protein formation is known as the amyloid hypothesis.

## Memory

Memory is one of the brain's most complex functions. Memory allows humans to recall a wide range of experiences and information, including recognition of other persons, names, events, feelings, visual impressions, language, sounds, taste sensations and more. The brain integrates these experiences, along with their associated emotions, into short- and long-term memories. The function of memory includes three components: encoding, storage, and retrieval. A defect in any link of this process can impair memory. Once processed, memories are held in short- and long-term "storage." Not everything in short-term memory is also consolidated into long-term memory. Repetition is one factor that increases the chances of a memory being transferred to long-term storage.

Until the middle of the twentieth century, many psychologists doubted that memory was a discrete function independent of the processes of language, movement or perception. One reason is that memory storage involves many different regions of the brain. Today it is known that these regions are not equally important. Many different types of memory storage exist, and certain regions of the brain are much more important for some types of storage than they are for other types (Kandel et al. 2000, 1228).

The neurosurgeon Wilder Penfield, another student of Charles Sherrington (who first mapped the activity of motor nerves), was the first person to obtain evidence that memory processes might be localized to specific regions of the human brain. By the 1940s, Penfield was able to apply electrical stimulation to map the motor, sensory, and language functions in the cerebral cortex of patients undergoing brain surgery for the treatment of epilepsy. Because the brain does not have brain receptors, patients are able to describe their impressions when different areas of the brain are stimulated.

One of Penfield's colleagues, the neurosurgeon Brenda Milner, demonstrated the effects on memory of bilateral (both sides) removal of portions of the temporal lobes in a 27-year-old patient called H.M. in case reviews. During surgery, the hippocampal formation, the amygdala, and parts of the multimodal association area of the temporal cortex were removed. Although his seizures stopped as a result of the procedure, the patient experienced a specific devastating memory deficit. He retained short-term memory for seconds or minutes and showed a good long-term recall of events that occurred before surgery. However, he was no longer able to transfer short-term memories into long-term memories (Penfield and Milner 1958, 475–77).

## Implicit, Explicit and Contextual Memory

Initially, Milner thought that bilateral medial temporal lobe lesions affected all aspects of memory. However, she found that even with profound memory deficits, affected patients are able to learn certain types of tasks, such as new motor skills, and they retain this information for as long as normal subjects do. Information regarding the performance of tasks is referred to as implicit or nondeclarative memory, which means that the information is recalled unconsciously. Explicit or declarative memory refers to factual knowledge of people, places and things. Highly flexible, explicit memory involves the association of multiple bits and pieces of information.

Implicit memory is more rigid and closely linked to the original stimulus conditions under which the learning occurred (Kandel et al. 2000, 1230). Motor skills and perception are examples of implicit memory. Implicit memory relies on regions of the brain that depend on stimuli, primarily the amygdala, the cerebellum and the basal ganglia in the reflex pathways. Implicit memory is associated with conditioning. Implicit memory is well preserved in aging individuals, including those in the early stages of AD. For this reason, in the early stages of AD, affected individuals are still able to complete learned tasks such as riding a bike.

Explicit memory allows individuals to unconsciously remember people, places, events, and facts. Explicit memory can be further classified as episodic or semantic. Episodic memory involves personal experiences or events, whereas semantic memory describes recollections that recognize facts such as music heard in the past. Semantic memory is used to store and later recall knowledge gleaned from teachers and books.

Contextual memory is the ability to remember how one knows something, or how to discern the origin of a specific memory. Contextual memory can include time, place, people involved, feelings, or any other kind of specific information related to the memory. Partial or erroneous processing of the contextual information may be due to time restraint, an impression of lesser importance, stress, distractions, or a deficit in information processing skills. Contextual memory is a basic step in the storing of long-term memories, which refers to the ability to remember emotional, social, spatial, or temporal circumstances related to an event.

## Practice Makes Perfect

Repetition and practice are the basic ways in which we store memories. To study this concept, Eric Kandel examined the cellular (and later the molecular) biology of memory, for which he received the Nobel Prize in 2000. By studying the giant marine snail Aplysia, Kandel demonstrated memory as a simple reflex response. The brain of Aplysia has very large neurons that make a small number of synaptic connections. These connections grew weaker or stronger in response to electrical stimuli. Rather than being fixed, these connections were plastic, although during development fixed connections existed for learning innate behaviors. Through learning, nervous systems are able to maintain flexible connections that store information as needed. These connections are strengthened through repetition of stimuli and tasks.

Various forms of learning, such as memory, forgetting, and thinking, are the result of synaptic contacts in different regions of the brain affected by the many different chemical messengers (neurotransmitters such as dopamine) contained in neurons. Aplysia exhibits both short- and long-term memory. Long-term memory in this species requires repeated training interspersed with periods of rest (Kandel 2018, 113).

In humans, short-term memory is limited to approximately 12 words or numbers. If these characters are not repeated, they are retained for only a few minutes. Long-term memory requires the synthesis of new proteins, which are required for establishing new neuronal connections. In this process, glial cells produce the essential fuel, which is lactate. For comparison, short-term memory is limited to working memory or random-access memory (RAM), whereas long-term memory can be compared to a computer's hard disk in which information is permanently stored. When emotionally significant, such as the events associated with an accident or trauma, memories can be stored immediately in long-term memory. In these circumstances, the amygdala is crucial for relaying the event to long-term memory storage. In post-traumatic stress disorders, the amygdala works too well, preventing the prefrontal cortex from signaling that the danger is over. An exaggerated response by the amygdala to negative stimuli also underlies borderline personality disorder, with symptoms of emotional instability and impulsiveness (Swaab 2014, 264).

Studies with human patients and experimental animals indicate that knowledge stored as explicit memory is first acquired through processing in the prefrontal, limbic, or parieto-occipital cortices that synthesize visual, auditory and somatic information. From there, the information is conveyed to the parahippocampal and perirhinal cortices, and then the entorhinal cortex, the dentate gyrus, the hippocampus, the subiculum, and finally back to the entorhinal cortex. From here, the information is relayed back to the parahippocampal and perirhinal cortices and ultimately back to the prefrontal, limbic or parieto-occipital cortices.

Defects in any of these structures can interfere with explicit memory storage. Different regions in the medial temporal lobe, however, can vary in their role in the process of memory. For instance, while the hippocampus is important for object recognition, damage to the perirhinal, parahippocampal, and entorhinal cortices produce greater deficits in memory storage. Lesions of the medial temporal lobe interfere only with the storage of new memories, meaning that affected patients may have good recall of earlier memories. This result suggests that the hippocampus is only a temporary way station for long-term memory.

Semantic memory is the type of long-term memory associated with the knowledge of objects, facts, and concepts, as well as words and their meaning. This includes the naming of objects, the definition of speech, and verbal fluency. Semantic knowledge is stored in a distributed fashion in the neocortex. Semantic knowledge is enforced through associations, such as similar information, over time. How well these associations have organized the information that we retain determines cognitive efficiency.

## Long-Term Memory Storage

During sleep the hippocampus constantly activates memories and transmits them to the cerebral cortex. Long-term memory storage starts in the entorhinal cortex after being briefly stored in the hippocampus in a process directed by the prefrontal cortex. The process has two pathways: (1) to the cerebral cortex for long-term storage and (2) arranging the information along the great arch of the fornex, suspended in the septum, to the hypothalamus, where some nerve fibers travel to the mammillary bods and some to the hypothalamus.

Because the entorhinal cortex is the first brain structure affected in Alzheimer's disease, deficits to long-term memory formation are one of the earliest symptoms.

Besides the amyloid plaque deposits, neurofibrillary tangles, and low cholinesterase levels seen in the brains of individuals with AD, the level of the protein clusterin is abnormally high in the brains of AD patients. Clusterin is known to interact with Aβ peptides to exacerbate the loss of tissue in the entorhinal cortex. Mutations in the clusterin gene are one of the risk factors for AD.

Problems with the storage of information in different areas of the brain cause different symptoms. Another early symptom in AD involves facial recognition, which is processed in the rear of the right hemisphere. In CAPGRAS syndrome or delusion, a patient is able to recognize friends, family members and acquaintances, although the patient feels no connection to the other person and becomes convinced that this person is an imposter.

The area of the brain considered the safest for memory storage is the remote memory, where language and music are stored. This area of the brain is the last to be affected in AD. Musical memory is presumably regulated by a subsystem of the long-term memory located on the side of the brain (parietal cortex). The visual cortex at the rear of the brain is also one of the last regions to be affected in AD. Visual artists with AD continue to have unimpaired artistic skills for long periods (Swaab 2014, 267).

While many of the symptoms in AD conform to a typical pattern beginning with long-term memory loss, specific brain changes associated with diet, nutrition, stress, and emotions contribute to the unique patient profile seen in individuals with AD.

## Summary

Since ancient times, scientists have attempted to decipher what defines consciousness and thought. While consciousness is still not fully understood, the cellular processes that produce thought are now well known. The brain's functional units called neurons are able to communicate with neurons in other areas of the nervous system to produce and control thoughts, learning, language, memory and movement.

The brain affected by Alzheimer's disease has been found to exhibit specific cellular changes, primarily cortical atrophy, extracellular amyloid beta protein deposits, intracellular neurofibrillary tangles, and a number of biochemical changes such as deficiencies of acetylcholine. These changes interfere with the ability of neurons to communicate with one another, thereby interfering with the formation and retrieval of memories and impressions that affect personality. Plaques initially form in the prefrontal cortex, a region involved in attention, self-control and problem solving. Neurofibrillary tangles start in the hippocampus. These plaques and tangles, along with acetylcholine deficiency, are thought to account for the early cognitive decline and memory loss seen in individuals with AD, although many individuals with normal cognitive function also exhibit these changes.

Over time, as more connections become damaged and neurons begin to die, regions such as the hippocampus begin to atrophy and the brain starts to lose crucial functions such as memory storage. As the disease progresses, symptoms related to memory become more obvious. Therapies directed at these changes, primarily therapies designed to reduce production of amyloid beta or increase production of acetylcholine, have not been successful in stopping the progression of the disease.

# Two

# Infection as a Primary Cause

This chapter describes the microbes that normally inhabit the human body and explains the ways in which infection, particularly infection affecting the central nervous system, can launch an inflammatory immune response that leads to the development of AD. Amyloid beta protein production and its processing from amyloid precursor protein are described to demonstrate how infection can lead to the increased amyloid beta plaques and neurofibrillary tangles seen in AD. Having discovered that amyloid beta protein is an antimicrobial agent, researchers are vigorously investigating the various microbes associated with AD. The amyloid beta protection hypothesis and the infectious disease theory of AD are included in this chapter.

## Microbes and Man

James Hill and his colleagues at Louisiana State University write, "Importantly, most of the changes seen in AD, such as inflammation, brain cell atrophy, immunological aberrations, amyloidogenesis, altered gene expression, and cognitive deficits are also seen as a consequence of microbial infection" (Hill et al. 2014). After all, the human body is home to approximately 10–100 trillion bacteria and other microscopic organisms. About one-tenth of our body's cells are human; the rest belong to the body's resident microorganisms (Kumar and Chordia 2017). These microorganisms, which are also known as microbes, are predominantly bacteria, archaea, fungi, spirochetes, and viruses (both latent and active), which are normally found in or on various sites of the human body, including the skin, nose, mouth, oral cavity, vagina and gut.

Referred to collectively as one's microbiota, these microorganisms' collection of genes is called the microbiome. The microbiome is an essential component of immunity that influences metabolism and modulates drug interactions, thereby contributing to human health. The human microbiome is a source of great genetic diversity, with no two human microbiomes being exactly the same. An individual's microbiome (described further in Chapter Three) contains about one hundred times more DNA than the individual's own human DNA.

The inhabitants of one's microbiota have important roles to play, such as facilitating digestion. They also produce a number of chemicals (including vitamins, neurotransmitters and hormones) and influence weight, food cravings and mood. Besides their more benign roles, they can adversely affect health when microbial strains become imbalanced, allowing an overgrowth of one microorganism, or when bacteria become attacked by viruses called bacteriophages. Infection occurs when microbes invade tissue, multiply, and cause a reaction in the host tissue. While only about 1 percent of bacteria cause infection, nearly all viruses are pathogenic (capable of causing disease). Regardless of their mode of attack, microbes exist to multiply, thrive, and find new hosts (Markel 2004, 16).

The immune system is a network of organs and cells designed to protect the human body from invasion by foreign or malignant cells. An innate immune response, usually involving inflammation, is the immune system's first line of defense against invasive pathogens, and it plays a crucial role in tissue regeneration and repair. A proper inflammatory response ensures the suitable resolution of inflammation and elimination of harmful stimuli. However, when the inflammatory reactions are inappropriate or chronic (persisting over a long period of time), they can affect and injure the tissue's surrounding normal cells.

Various infections have long been known to cause conditions of dementia. These include syphilis, neuroborreliosis, tuberculosis and meningitis. When Alois Alzheimer studied the brain tissue of Auguste Deter (later described as the first patient with Alzheimer's disease), he initially suspected that an infection was the underlying cause of her dementia. However, his supervisor, Emil Kraepelin, urged Alzheimer to present his case report as though his patient had a new disease, ignoring the obvious signs of tuberculosis, which included excessive weight loss and what Sir Thomas Clouston, the superintendent of the prestigious Royal Edinburgh Asylum, called the "monomania of suspicion" (Broxmeyer 2016, ix).

Clouston wrote that the "monomania of suspicion" nearly always occurs in patients who die of central nervous system tuberculosis. With regard to patients with tuberculosis who developed dementia, Clouston remarked that this was the most dreaded event that could happen and occurred in about 30 percent of central nervous system tuberculosis cases. Clouston was amazed at the lengths to which Alzheimer and Kraepelin went to totally ignore the obvious signs of tuberculosis (Broxmeyer 2016, ix). A thorough description of the other studies that supported a diagnosis of tuberculosis in Auguste Deter can be found in Lawrence Broxmeyer's extremely well-researched book, *Alzheimer's Disease: How its Bacterial Cause Was Found and Then Discarded.*

In the last three decades, with the discovery of other infections—such as the prion diseases, human immunodeficiency virus, and the *Herpes simplex* virus—that can cause dementia, along with the fact that inflammation in the brain (neuroinflammation) is another characteristic finding in AD, the role of infection as a preventable cause of AD has entered the diagnostic arena, particularly in cases of late-onset AD (LOAD). In addition, because the amyloid beta (Aβ) protein has been found to have antimicrobial properties, the role of infection in AD has become even more evident. This chapter describes the infectious disease theory and the antimicrobial protection hypothesis, along with considerable evidence that supports the role of infection in the development of AD.

## The Antimicrobial Properties of the Amyloid Beta Protein

The amyloid deposit Aβ protein is a subunit protein or fragment derived from its precursor, amyloid precursor protein (APP), through a process known as proteolytic processing. In this process, the enzymes beta and gamma secretase cause APP to split into uneven fragments. The slightly longer variant with 42 amino acids is directly toxic to nerve cells. In this case, Aβ appears to stimulate the release of oxygen free radicals, triggering a destructive biochemical cascade in the brain.

While it affects neurons in specific areas of the brain in AD, Aβ is produced by all of the body's cells during normal metabolism and as a protective step in the immune system's response to infection, trauma and brain injury. Bacteria inhabiting the gastrointestinal tract produce numerous chemicals, including amyloid protein.

It has also long been known that Aβ may have either neurotrophic or neurotoxic effects depending on neuronal age, protein concentration, and the presence of fetal or adult neurons. Amyloid plaques are not diagnostic for AD because they are found in the brains of individuals with many disorders, including Alzheimer's disease, Huntington's disease, type 2 diabetes, secondary amyloidosis, brain infections, and prion diseases. These diseases all demonstrate marked inflammation at the sites of Aβ deposits. These deposits are known to injure the surrounding tissue and impair the ability of neurons to communicate with one another.

Aβ protein molecules are sticky proteins containing up to 43 amino acid

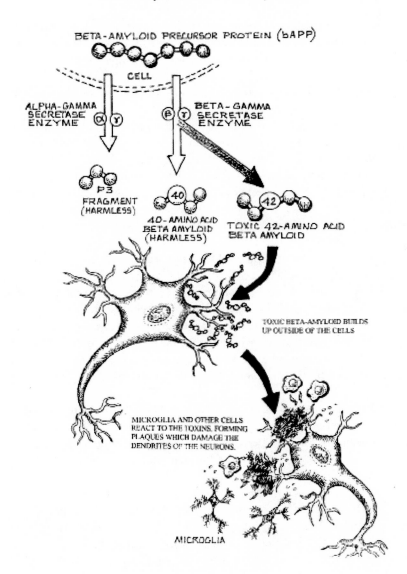

**Amyloid Plaque Formation.**

residues. Neurotrophic effects (that is, effects beneficial to neurons) may reside in the first 28 residues of Aβ since there is evidence of neurite (neuron extensions—that is, axons and dendrites) outgrowth as well as neuronal survival in these shorter forms. The neurotoxic effects seen in the longer residues include increases in intracellular calcium, increases in induced cell destruction via increased apoptosis (programmed cell death), activated microglia, enhanced oxidation, increased excitotoxicity, and hypoglycemic damage.

Before the development of neurofibrillary tangles in AD, Aβ is found to aggregate between neurons and form diffuse deposits as well as amyloid cores in the brains of patients with AD. Senile neuritic plaques in AD consist of Aβ protein cores surrounded by activated microglia (indicating an immune system response), fibrillary astrocytes, and dystrophic or abnormal neuritis (neuron inflammation). The type of Aβ seen in senile plaques has 42 amino acids and exerts neurotoxic effects, causing neuronal destruction. High levels of toxic Aβ are also associated with reduced levels of the neurotransmitter acetylcholine and are suspected of disrupting channels that carry the elements sodium, potassium and calcium. These elements serve the brain as ions, producing electric charges that must fire regularly in order for signals to pass from one nerve cell to another. If the neuron channels that carry ions are damaged, the resulting imbalance can interfere with nerve function and signal transmission.

Despite their obvious role in AD, these deposits are also seen in normal aging, suggesting that it is the maturation or density of plaque deposits, the toxicity of early forms (Aβ oligomers) or shifts in the pathways that produce or remove Aβ that are critical to AD development. The notion that AD is directly caused by increased Aβ formation is known as the amyloid hypothesis. For many years, AD therapies have focused on reducing production of Aβ. To date, none of these therapies have proven successful, and in trials of treatments aimed at reducing Aβ, an increased rate of infections was seen.

While many metabolic factors may contribute to Alzheimer's disease, the role of infection is proving to be the most plausible. For the first time, a new symposium, "Role of Microbes in the Development of Alzheimer's Disease: State of the Art," headlined the International Association of Gerontology and Geriatrics (IAGG) conference in San Francisco on July 24, 2017. Here hundreds of scientists participated and spoke with the presenters after the lectures. The symposium provided an alternative approach to understanding how potential microbial infection and a corresponding innate immune response lead to the destruction of neurons and synapses in AD (Fülöp et al. 2018, "Role of Microbes"). The following section provides a summary of the main topics presented at this conference.

At the IAGG conference, five researchers presented their results on the role of infection in AD. Professor Ruth Itzhaki presented her work on viruses, specifically *Herpes simplex* virus-1 (HSV-1), based on experimental evidence from AD brains and infected cell cultures. (The findings of Itzhaki and the other speakers are described in Chapters Six through Nine.)

Professor Judith Miklossy presented research on the high prevalence of bacterial infections that correlate with AD, specifically spirochete infections, which have long been known to cause dementia (in cases of syphilis). She demonstrated how spirochetes drive senile plaque formation and how plaque is, in fact, a bacterial biofilm.

A biofilm is a polysaccharide, protein, nucleic acid conglomerate secreted by one microorganism or by an entire microbial community working together, which is held together with amyloid protein. A biofilm surrounds the microorganism that secreted it and protects it from antimicrobial agents and immune attack. Even when a biofilm is attacked with a solution of Lysol, some microorganisms are destroyed while others continue to multiply. In the case of some microbes such as *Clostridium botulinum* (which causes botulism), the microbe has the ability to hibernate and form a tough cell wall cladding called an endospore to help resist environmental stresses. The hardiest known form of life on earth, an endospore can be built within hours (Bone 2018, 24).

Also presenting a report at the symposium, Professor Brian Balin described the involvement of brain tissue infected by the *Chlamydia pneumoniae* (*C. pneumoniae*) bacterium and its associated innate immune system response, which results in the initiation of tissue damage. In his study, Balin and his team identified this organism in 17 of 19 postmortem brain tissue specimens from patients with AD. In the control group, the researchers only found one sample with *C. pneumoniae*. In the affected AD brains, the infection was localized to brain areas connected to olfaction (sense of smell), such as the amygdala and entorhinal cortex, and also the hippocampus proper and temporal and frontal cortices. All cell types (neurons, astrocytes, microglia, and endothelial) tissue cells were infected to some extent. The researchers proposed that infection occurred through the respiratory tract and noted that early symptoms in AD include a loss of the sense of smell.

Representing his laboratory at the Research Center on Aging at the University of Sherbrooke in Quebec, Professor Támas Fülöp described how AD-associated Aβ is an antibacterial, antifungal and antiviral innate immune effector that is produced in reaction to microorganisms that attack the brain. His study focused on the role of Aβ in infections with viruses that have envelopes, particularly *Herpes simplex* virus-1 (HSV-1). The researchers found that Aβ was effective against the enveloped viruses influenza and HSV-1 but not against adenovirus, which does not possess an envelope. In addition, the researchers described their finding that beta-secretase enzyme activation was the origin of the increased Aβ production. Inhibition of this enzyme likewise inhibited Aβ production.

Professor Annelise Barron described her experiments showing that there is strong sequence-specific binding between the AD-associated Aβ and another innate immune effector, the peptide LL-37. Chronic underexpression (causing deficiencies) of LL-37 could be the factor that both allows chronic infection in brain tissue and facilitates the pathological accumulations of Aβ.

## Antimicrobial Proteins and Peptides

The ability to produce antimicrobial proteins and peptides is an important contribution to host defense in humans and other multicellular animals. The larger antimicrobial proteins, which contain more than 100 amino acids, often contain enzymes capable of lysing and destroying microbes or that bind with nutrients needed for microbe survival. The smaller antimicrobial peptides primarily act to disrupt the structure or function of microbial cell membranes. Some of these peptides are produced constitutively while others are produced in response to infection or inflammation (Ganz 2013).

The putative roles of Aβ include providing protection from infections, repairing leaks in the blood-brain barrier, promoting recovery from injury, and regulating synaptic function. Studies show that the cellular production of Aβ increases quickly in response to a physiological challenge and generally diminishes upon recovery. Normally present in a soluble form, Aβ is secreted in the extracellular spaces of the brain and then rapidly cleared by the cerebrospinal fluid (CSF) and the vascular system (Brothers et al. 2018).

The highest antimicrobial peptide concentrations are found in animal tissues that are exposed to microbes or in cells that are involved in host defense. Research suggests that antimicrobial peptides released as a response to infection can activate the adaptive immune system by attracting antigen-presenting dendritic cells to the site of invasion, which is one of the first steps in the immune response. LL-37, which is also known as CAP-18 (for cathelicidin antimicrobial peptide), is a gene encoding for the only member of the human cathelicidin family, a family of antimicrobial peptides normally found in macrophages as well as polymorphonuclear white blood cells. The strength of many other antimicrobial peptides is characterized by comparison to the innate immune effector LL-37.

Recent evidence based on initial research conducted by Harvard's Robert Moir indicates that Aβ is an antimicrobial peptide that influences amyloid beta precursor protein (APP) processing in a way that produces more Aβ oligomers (as fibrillary aggregates) in an effort to protect the host from various infectious agents. These soluble oligomers can go on to form structured proto fibrils that entrap pathogens and disrupt cell membranes. These early aggregates are considered more toxic than Aβ in neuropathic diseases and are especially toxic to synapses (Chiti and Dobson 2006; Monsonego et al. 2013).

With eventual production and overproduction of Aβ, patients have increased resistance to infection from both bacteria and viruses (Gosztyla et al. 2018). Aβ has been shown to possess antimicrobial activity against numerous microbes. In one study comparing Aβ to LL-37 in *Herpes simplex* virus-1, Influenza A, *Enterococcus faecalis*, *Escherichia coli*, *Listeria monocytogenes*, *Salmonella typhimurium*, *Staphylococcus aureus*, *Staphylococcus epidermis*, *Streptococcus pneumoniae* and *Candida albicans*, Aβ proved to have antimicrobial activity against all of these microbes, and its potency was equal to or exceeding that of LL-37 in seven of eight bacteria (Gosztyla et al. 2018).

Studies showing that the presence of Aβ in nematodes infected with *Candida albicans* is associated with reduced mortality demonstrated that Aβ also functions as an antimicrobial peptide in lower life forms. In humans, Aβ confers immune resistance in the human innate immune system. That is, the innate immune system creates antimicrobial peptides, which, along with innate immune cells, form the body's first line of defense upon recognizing infectious agents. However, over time in chronic, severe or untreated infections, the continuous production of Aβ can contribute to deposits of insoluble Aβ plaque formation characterized by insoluble misfolded proteins and biofilms. Misfolded Aβ proteins are the result of a transition from alpha helix to beta sheets, which characterize amyloid deposits in AD.

Aβ is produced in the brain by astrocytes and neurons. In the skin, skeletal muscle and intestinal tissue, the epithelial cells that make up these tissues secrete Aβ. In the brain, the normal soluble form of Aβ is first secreted in extracellular spaces between neurons and then rapidly cleared by the cerebrospinal fluid and vascular system within two hours. After it is cleared, Aβ is removed from the circulation system by the capillary beds of the kidneys, liver, gastrointestinal tract, and skin. The most abundant type of Aβ in the brain is 40 amino acids long, while the second most common isoform is 42 amino acids long (Brothers et al. 2018). When Aβ forms insoluble fibrils, the fibrils aggregate with other Aβ molecules to form β-pleated sheets of insoluble plaque deposits. Aβ oligomers and fibrils that do not form plaque are cleared very slowly from the circulation system.

## Curli Fibrils

The topic of curli fibrils provides additional evidence as to the role of infection in AD. Curli fibrils (amyloid proteins that were first discovered in the late 1980s) are fiber-like structures consisting of curli proteins that allow bacteria to stick to host tissue and to each other and form colonies. Curli fibrils are morphologically identical to amyloid fibrils found in AD. Both curli proteins, which can enter the brain via leaky gut syndrome, and amyloid beta plaque deposits lead to increased production of Aβ. Because of the unique resemblance of curli proteins to amyloid beta fibers, researchers believe that Alzheimer's plaques may resemble colonies of bacteria, which would result in the chronic inflammation and Aβ production seen in AD.

Researchers at the University of California, Davis, have found that amyloid beta plaques and certain gut bacteria elicit the same response by human immune cells. Andreas Bäumler, a professor of microbiology and medical immunology at UC Davis, showed that the immune systems of mice injected with *Escherichia coli* and *Salmonella* are triggered by curli fibrils produced by many species of *Enterobacteriaceae*.

In their animal study on mice, Bäumler and his colleagues discovered that the immune response to curli fibrils is controlled by a protein called toll-like receptor 2 (TLR2). TLR2 is expressed on the surface of certain cells that pass on appropriate signals to the immune system. The researchers found that the mechanism involving TLR2 was triggered by the major curli fibril protein CsgA and by amyloid beta, but only when these proteins were allowed to aggregate into amyloids. Their research goal is to find a substance that inhibits TLR2, which would reduce Aβ production in AD regardless of whether bacterial infection was present (UC Davis 2009).

## APP Processing and Aβ

The production of Aβ occurs in a process in which peptides are cleaved from amyloid precursor protein (APP). APP, which is also known as amyloid beta precursor protein, is the parent transmembrane protein from which Aβ protein is derived. Its expression or presence is stimulated by endogenous factors such as cytokines (immune system chemicals including growth factors), estrogens, head trauma and excitotoxicity. Increases in this precursor protein occur at the same time that neurons begin to differentiate (into specialized neurons with specific functions that eventually migrate into different parts of the central nervous system).

The cloning of the gene mutation coding for APP on chromosome 21 led to an understanding of the role of genes in conferring susceptibility to AD (a topic described in Chapter Eleven). APP can exist in different isoforms derived from alternative mRNA gene splicing. These gene products are expressed in different tissues, with the highest concentrations occurring in the brain.

APP occurs in cells throughout the body, including the gastrointestinal tract, where it is processed by bacteria. In the brain, APP is produced by astrocytes and neurons. In the first step of APP cleavage, the beta-site APP cleaving enzyme (BACE1), which is the major beta secretase enzyme in the brain, cleaves APP to release the C99 fragment of APP. This fragment gives rise to various species of Aβ peptide during subsequent cleavage by alpha- and gamma-secretase enzymes. A multi-protein complex that includes presenilin 1 or 2, nicastrin, presenilin enhancer 2, and anterior pharynx defective 1 regulates gamma secretase activity. Studies have demonstrated that inhibiting beta- or gamma-secretase enzymes or enhancing alpha-secretase enzymes reduces Aβ production (Chow et al. 2010).

When alpha-secretase cleaves APP, secreted APP alpha (sAPPα) is generated in a process called shedding. This production is considered beneficial to neurons due to its ability to protect against glucose deprivation and excitotoxicity. It accomplishes this by decreasing calcium channels and increasing potassium currents, thereby stabilizing the resting membrane potential.

APP is a dependence receptor, that is, a protein with three primary isoforms occurring in AD, which are restricted to the central nervous system. These forms arise from alternative splicing, depending on their length in amino acid, (i.e. APP695, APP751 and APP770). As transmembrane receptors these isoforms lie on the neuron's outer surface and appear to stick out of neurons. Proteolysis of APP by alpha or beta secretase enzymes causes the secretion of soluble peptides, designated as sAPP isoforms.

When APP is cut at three spots by caspase and beta and gamma secretase enzymes, it produces four peptides: secreted APP beta (sAPPβ), Jcasp, C32, and amyloid beta (Aβ). Beta-secretase activity is mediated by the BACE1 enzyme and cleaves APP to form sAPPβ, a protein that lacks the benefits of the alpha fragment. It is associated with activation of the caspase 6 enzyme, which causes disintegration of neuronal axons. The other three peptides—Jcasp (or AICD), C32, and Aβ—all contribute to the destruction of neurons and synapses in AD.

Depending on which secretase enzymes initiate the process and whether two or four peptides are produced, Aβ protein may exist as a harmless peptide chain or a longer form with more amino acids and the propensity to damage neurons and form plaque. As a dependence receptor, APP helps regulate programmed cell death or apoptosis. When Aβ is produced, it acts as an anti-trophin by binding to APP and preventing trophic signaling, which controls cell death. Too much binding blocks the receptor, which tells too many neurons to die. The most common form of Aβ is Aβ1-40 (with 40 amino acids), and the most toxic form is Aβ1-42 (with 42 amino acids).

Secreted, soluble Aβ can bind to other molecules of Aβ to form oligomers (complex of molecules with a limited number of repeating units) in the extracellular spaces between neurons that are cleared more slowly from the brain. These oligomers have potent, broad-spectrum antimicrobial properties by forming insoluble fibrils that entrap pathogens and disrupt cell membranes, conferring resistance to infection. However, with continuous production, these oligomers (which can be more toxic than Aβ) can inhibit synaptic transmission and ultimately cause neuronal spine and synapse loss. They can also accumulate to form insoluble Aβ plaques. Plaques known as Aβ dimers, which are produced by the Aβ fragments with 40–42 amino acids, have been shown to be the most potent form of Aβ oligomers.

The toxicity of oligomers appears to stem from their misfolded proteins. When proteins are converted from their soluble native state into soluble oligomers, a wide range of non-native species is generated, including many with misfolded protein molecules. These molecules inevitably expose on their surfaces an array of molecules that are normally buried within the peptide bonds. The non-native character of misfolded proteins likely triggers aberrant events as the molecules interact with cellular components such as cell membranes, ultimately leading to neuronal cell death (Chiti and Dobson 2006). The misfolded protein oligomers form insoluble fibrils and eventually form Aβ molecules with a misfolded protein nature.

## Influences on APP Processing

While secretase enzymes, which are under the influence of genes, are important factors in determining the specific pathway that APP will take, Dale Bredesen, MD, describes the process as dependent on the specific molecule to which APP binds. If APP binds to a molecule called netrin-1, APP is cut at one site, and two beneficial fragments are produced. If APP binds with Aβ, APP is cut at three sites, resulting in the production of three fragments of amyloid beta. Together, APP and Aβ form what Bredesen calls a prionic loop, with the process continuing, producing more neuron- and synapse-destroying Aβ (Bredesen 2017, 74).

Bredesen reports that APP is known to respond to a number of different molecules that influence the production of the more benign products of APP cleavage. These molecules include adequate thyroid hormone, estrogen, testosterone, insulin, the cytokine nuclear factor-kappa beta (NF-κβ) and the longevity-associated protein sirtuin SIRT1 (which is described further in Chapter Twelve). Bredesen has developed a diagnostic protocol that enables him to screen for treatable disorders such as hypothyroidism; diabetes; Lyme disease; adrenal disease; deficiencies of vitamins B12, B1 and D; and numerous other diseases. With appropriate treatment, Bredesen is able to affect APP processing so that more benign forms of Aβ are produced.

Bredesen's protocol includes screening for endocrine and metabolic disorders, as well as nutrient and mineral deficiencies that contribute to the production of Aβ and cause neurological symptoms that can be reversed with treatment. Some test results can suggest problems in other areas and require additional tests. For instance, Bredesen describes an abnormally low ratio of zinc to copper (that is, lower than the normal ratio of 1:1) as a risk factor for Alzheimer's disease. A high level of copper relative to zinc, which occurs when the zinc-to-copper ratio is low, is a common finding in hypothyroidism and suggests the need for a full thyroid panel with appropriate tests for TSH receptor antibodies, which can falsely lower the TSH level.

## Neurofibrillary Tangles

Tau protein is normally found inside neurons and serves to stabilize microtubules. Tau protein is abundant in the central nervous system, although it is less prominent in astrocytes and oligodendrocytes than in neurons. Tau protein is also less commonly seen in other parts of the body. In general, proteins need to have a three-dimensional shape to function properly. This shape is maintained by folding, a process in which the amino acids that make up the protein twist themselves. When a molecular defect results in misfolding of tau protein, toxic clumps are formed, which create neurofibrillary tangles. Neurofibrillary tangles interfere with the ability of neurons to send signals.

## The Postmortem Brain

The brains of individuals with AD or related disorders who participate in clinical studies and donate their bodies to science after their death are stored in brain banks. Researchers use these brain specimens for postmortem studies. Locations of brain banks throughout the world can be found at www.alzforum.org/brain-banks.

Senile Aβ-rich plaques in postmortem specimens from AD patients are frequently strewn with microbial, fungal or viral DNA. The outer surface of plaque in the postmortem brain can also be coated with a biofilm. Bacteria have the property of quorum sensing, which gives them the ability to sense their number. When they reach a certain number, they can aggregate together, sometimes with other microorganisms, to form a biofilm, which increases their microbial activity and makes them more resistant to destruction (Bone 2018, 229).

The majority of cases of AD are sporadic, with less than 5 percent of cases having an early onset of the disease (EOAD). Less than 2 percent of cases of EOAD are related to autosomal dominant genetic mutations (Alonso et al. 2018). Aging and the APOE-ε4 gene allele are the main risk factors for AD in patients older than 65 years, although most individuals with this gene mutation do not go on to develop AD. The APOE-ε4 mutation is responsible for around 17 percent of all AD cases among the elderly (Swaab 2014, 339), suggesting that other causes are involved. Postmortem studies show that microbial infection of the brain is very common in AD, and it is more common in individuals who have the APOE-ε4 genetic mutation.

Studies show that compared to age-matched controls, patients with AD were more likely to have fungi belonging to the genuses *Fusarium, Alternaria, Botyris, Candida,* and *Malassezia*. Fungal infection is frequently accompanied by bacterial infection. *Proteobacteria* was the most prominent bacteria in both patient and control brains, whereas *Burkholderiaceae, Chlamydia pneumoniae,* and *Staphylococcaceae* exhibited higher percentages in AD patients than in controls (Alonso et al. 2018). Ruth Itzhaki and her colleagues have found a number of viruses, particularly herpes viruses, present in postmortem AD brain studies (Itzhaki et al. 2016; Itzhaki and Lathe 2018).

Microglial cells are the brain's primary immune cells. In AD patients, markers of microglial activation are increased when compared to control patients. The presence of activated microglial cells in postmortem brain samples from AD patients provides additional evidence that microbial infection and its resulting inflammation lead to the development of AD (Hopperton et al. 2018). The immune response and the changes that are seen in patients with AD are described further in Chapter Four.

In addition to the presence of microbes in the brains of AD patients, systemic inflammation is frequently observed. This effect is manifested by elevations in pro-inflammatory cytokines and markers of inflammation (such as C-reactive protein), and the presence of complement components in amyloid plaques.

Besides obvious infections such as periodontitis from oral treponemes and various herpes viruses that are associated with AD, intestinal bacteria can also infect the brain. Intestinal microorganisms are likewise known to produce Aβ protein, which can enter the brain through leaky gut syndrome (described in Chapter Three), and defects in the blood-brain barrier (described in Chapter Five) can add to the neuronal damage that occurs in AD.

## *The Infection Hypothesis*

The brain in AD has two main pathological characteristics: the presence of extracellular Aβ plaques and intraneuronal neurofibrillary tangles (NFTs) formed by tau protein. However, these characteristics are not unique to AD. Other disorders of the central nervous system including chronic infections develop with the production of these same hallmarks. In addition, the discovery of the antimicrobial properties of Aβ suggests that infections may result in deposits of Aβ in the brain (Sochocka et al. 2017).

Current data also suggest that vascular factors, oxidative stress and a process of neuroinflammation in the brain are primary contributors to AD development. Therefore, the immune response to infection and the development of inflammation are early steps in the process that leads to AD. An inappropriate response, which is more common in aging individuals and those with nutrient abnormalities (such as increased iron or low vitamin D), can alter the blood-brain barrier and cause an increased production of pro-inflammatory cytokines and other immune system mediators.

While acute inflammation promotes healing, chronic inflammation, which is usually low grade but persistent, elicits an immune response that supports the destruction of neurons and their synapses. Matrix metalloproteinases (MMPs), a branch of the large family of metalloproteinases, are also thought to be involved in the pathology of several neurodegenerative disorders, including AD. As enzymes, MMPs are activated by inflammatory mediators or by peptide aggregates such as Aβ deposits. Normally, MMPs help repair tissues, but when they are continuously activated, they contribute to neuronal destruction. High levels of MMPs in cerebrospinal fluid (CSF) are considered early indicators of AD (Sochocka et al. 2017). As with other early markers (including Aβ), high levels are seen in the CSF early on, before symptoms develop, with declining CSF levels as the disease progresses. In blood, high levels of Aβ are seen in the mild cognitive impairment (MCI) stage of AD, with steadily declining levels as the disease progresses.

According to the infection hypothesis, reactivation of viruses and chronic infections with other microorganisms affect the same areas of the brain that are targeted in infection with the human herpes virus (HHV-1), which affects about 80 percent of the population. Like most latent viruses, HHV-1 can be reactivated when the immune system is weak due to various diseases or as a consequence of aging (Sochocka et al. 2017). While viral reactivation or reactivation in persistent bacterial infections may not cause noticeable symptoms, viral and bacterial reactivation causes a persistent immune response, especially in individuals with the APOE-ε4 mutation.

The higher permeability of the blood-brain barrier over the hypothalamus in the elderly, as well as their greater risk for reactivation of hepatitis C, *Cytomegalovirus*, and *Herpes zoster* (shingles), increases their risk for this heightened immune response. The infection hypothesis is also supported by the fact that a number of studies show that standard antiviral drugs inhibit the pathological changes observed in AD that are associated with viral infections. (It should be noted that antiviral drugs also inhibit the activity of some bacteria.)

Ruth Itzhaki and her colleagues were the first to identify *Herpes simplex* virus-1 (HSV-1) as a causative factor in AD since it clearly infects the brain and has the ability to directly cause the production of toxic Aβ and the hyperphosphorylation of tau protein that leads to neurofibrillary tangles (Fülöp et al. 2018, "Infection Hypothesis").

Marta Sochocka and her colleagues report that of the bacteria studied in AD, *Chlamydia pneumoniae* is considered the most plausible infectious agent because it is known to infect all of the brain's cells, including endothelial cells, astrocytes, microglial cells, and neurons. In addition, *C. pneumoniae* may reside in an intracellular inclusion that resists lysosomal fusion and immune regulation. Because these bacteria require nutrients from the host, they are able to manipulate the host cell as well as the immune response. With persistent infection, there is constant interaction between microglial cells in the brain that regulate the immune response and neurons (Sochocka et al. 2017).

## The Antimicrobial Protection Hypothesis

Similar to the infection hypothesis of AD, the antimicrobial protection hypothesis explains that ongoing innate immune-mediated inflammation triggered by the presence of antimicrobial amyloid beta peptide causes the continual production of amyloid beta plaque seen in AD.

Genetic mutations lead to Aβ production in early-onset familial Alzheimer's disease, a condition representing less than 1 percent of all cases of AD and occurring in a limited number of families. While early-onset Alzheimer's disease (EOAD) represents less than 5 percent of all cases, many individuals with EOAD do not have the deterministic genes seen in the familial cases. These individuals may, however, have genes that have yet to be associated with AD. The majority of patients who have the sporadic form of AD show evidence of the normal Aβ production that occurs in older individuals, making some researchers regard AD as an accelerated form of aging.

According to Harvard professor Robert Moir and his team, early deposits of Aβ are generated as an innate immune response to genuine or mistakenly perceived challenges to the immune system. In the first step of the immune response, Aβ in the brain entraps and neutralizes infectious pathogens. As Aβ forms soluble oligomers and insoluble fibrils, this process triggers the immune system pathways in the brain that help fight infection and clear Aβ deposits. However, an increased microbial burden within the brain directly exacerbates Aβ production, neuroinflammation, and AD progression (Moir et al. 2018).

Rather than junk molecules clogging up the brain, amyloid beta protein has a very important role and is one of the top most-conserved proteins in all of biology. Its antimicrobial properties alone make it capable of being conserved and passed down for 400 million years (Proal 2017).

Evidence demonstrates that amyloid beta oligomers have potent, broad-spectrum antimicrobial properties by forming fibrils capable of entrapping pathogens and disrupting cell membranes. Overexpression of Aβ confers increased resistance to infection from both bacteria and viruses. The antimicrobial role of Aβ may explain why patients in clinical trials for compounds that deplete Aβ have a high rate of infections (Gosztyla et al. 2018).

According to the antimicrobial protection hypothesis, cognitive decline in AD patients is not correlated with the levels of senile plaque formation or insoluble Aβ. These observations suggest the existence of soluble toxic forms of Aβ, which have been identified as soluble Aβ oligomers derived from soluble monomers and insoluble Aβ aggregates. These oligomers, which are found in high numbers in the brains of AD patients, cause synaptic and cognitive dysfunction in vivo (within the body) and synapse loss and neuronal death in vitro (test tube studies). The production of senile plaque is thought to occur in order to protect neurons from the toxicity of diffusible Aβ oligomers.

Disruptions in lipid levels have also been observed in AD and may be related to the production of lipid particles (particularly lipopolysaccharides) by microorganisms. The biochemical alterations seen in AD related to perturbations in gut flora are described in Chapter Three.

## Summary

Numerous studies conducted over the past twenty years have shown that brain infection is a common finding in patients with AD. Many different microbes, including fungi, bacteria, spirochetes, virus, and protozoa, have been identified in the postmortem brain specimens from AD patients and, to a lesser extent, in control subjects.

With the discovery that Aβ is an antimicrobial peptide, and the realization that Aβ protein is produced in response to infection as part of the innate immune response, the focus on infection and the immune system's response as causes of AD has come to the forefront. During the immune response (which is stimulated by both infection and the presence of Aβ), toxic, soluble Aβ oligomers are formed. These oligomers contribute to the destruction of neurons and their synaptic connections. The presence of the APOE-ε4 is seen more frequently in individuals with brain infections, and disruptions in lipid metabolism are suspected of being a contributing factor. There is no one infectious agent considered responsible for all cases of AD. Rather, a number of infectious agents (including the *Mycobacterium* species suspected of being present in the first Alzheimer's patient) are capable of causing the neuroinflammation and neurodegenerative changes that lead to a loss of cognitive function.

# THREE

# Microorganisms and the Microbiome

Detailed studies of ancient rocks embedded in the Earth's crust provide clues about the planet's age. Based on these studies, researchers estimate that what is known as Earth emerged around 4.54 billion years (Redd 2019). Into this watery world, Eugenia Bone writes, the earth's first life forms emerged approximately 3.8 billion years ago (Bone 2018, 20). Animals first appeared on Earth between 900 and 650 million years ago. In their present form, humans (Homo sapiens) have existed for approximately 100,000 years.

This chapter serves as an introduction to the trillions of microbes that coexist with humans. From a medical standpoint, the following pages describe the paradox of microbial life—specifically how microorganisms are essential for life processes and how they can cause disease. Microorganisms belong to the two major classes of living organisms: the prokaryotes and the eukaryotes (which include humans). A description of the basic cells in these classifications is included. As the basis of life, the cell is present in all living organisms, and the basic cell structure is the same regardless of whether the cell belongs to a eukaryote worm or a neuron.

In the sections on the microbiome, readers are introduced to the majority of genetic information stored in the human body from the microbiome, which is contained in the DNA that exists in one's personal microbial inventory, the microbiota. In addition, this chapter offers insight into the ways in which microbes normally present in the gut or oral cavity can be introduced into the central nervous system, where they cause a number of biochemical changes consistent with the clinical picture in Alzheimer's disease. Alterations to the gut microbe that are routinely seen in individuals with AD add more supporting evidence to the role of infection in the disease process. The role of microbes in switching genes on and off is also described in the section on epigenetics.

## Microbiota and Microbiome

The microbiota is an individual's unique ecological community of commensal, mutual, and pathogenic microorganisms found inside, on, and around all multicellular organisms from plants to animals. A human's microbiota includes bacteria, archaea, protozoa, fungi and viruses. If humans and microbes interact in a way that benefits both parties, this arrangement is called mutualism. If in this interaction one species benefits and the other remains neutral or unaffected, this is called commensalism. For instance, commensalism occurs when microbes in our gut digest the harmful sugars in breast milk that a newborn can't digest. However, if one species in the interaction benefits to the detriment of the other, this is called parasitism, and it can lead to pathogenic diseases. The microbes responsible for disease are called pathogens (Dietert 2016, 33–34).

The human colon alone is colonized with approximately 10–100 trillion microbes with a total weight of around three pounds. Each individual's gut microbiota is unique and offers clues to predisposing diseases. For instances, individuals with type 2 diabetes have increased blood levels of bacterial 16S rDNA (high levels of bacteria) from their gut microbiota long before the disease develops (Serino et al. 2012).

While the words *microbiome* and *microbiota* are often used interchangeably, *microbiome* refers to all of the genetic material present in an organism's microbiota. The microbiome is a composite of all microorganisms that reside on and within the human body, including the skin, oral and nasal mucosa, and the urogenital and gastrointestinal tracts. An individual's microbiome is influenced by diet, as well as the air they breathe; the soil and dirt they touch or ingest; the countries they travel to; the antibiotics and other medicines they take; their family members; family pets, which help in sharing the microbiota of family members; the pesticides and toxins they inadvertently ingest; and many other environmental factors. While family members do not share the same microbiota, they do have similar microbiomes.

Alterations to the gut microbiota that damage its normal balance, interfere with microbial processes, and injure the gut membrane have a profound effect on health and are associated with a number of different neurodegenerative diseases, including AD. The biochemical changes that occur in AD when there are alterations to the gut microbiome causing conditions of dysbiosis are described later in this chapter. The effects of these changes on the immune system and its response are described in Chapter Four.

### Life Forms

The first microbes on Earth reported to exist are the tiny archaea and a species of bacteria now recognized as *Cyanobacteria*. Microbes exist in two basic forms: acellular (that is, lacking a cellular structure) microbes (which are also called infectious particles) and cellular microbes with contents contained within a cell wall or membrane. Cellular microbes are also known as microorganisms.

The first life forms, the prokaryotes (along with the eukaryote microorganisms that emerged later), are essential for the existence of plant and animal life. For instance, the presence of fungi in soil facilitates the absorption of nutrients in plants that share the soil. Microorganisms can also cause bodily harm when their presence leads to infection or when chemicals released by microbes cause microbial intoxication (for instance, in *Staphylococcal* food poisoning).

## Prokaryotes—Bacteria and Archaea

Depending on differences in the structure of certain ribosomal ribonucleic acid (rRNA) molecules, living entities are classified as either prokaryotes or eukaryotes. However, viruses, while able to survive and replicate, are neither prokaryotes nor eukaryotes.

The first forms of life—and the majority of life forms on Earth today—are the prokaryotes, which existed long before animals, fungi and plants emerged. Prokaryotes are members of the Kingdom *Prokaryotae* or *Monera*. Although they do not have nuclei, prokaryotes (which include the families of bacteria and archaea) consist of a primary mass of DNA and one or more secondary threads or rings of DNA called plasmids.

Prokaryotes also contain ribosomes and a chromosome and are able to move, although they do not have mouths, stomachs, or anuses. Nutrients diffuse in and out through their cell membranes. Extremely small, hundreds of thousands of prokaryotes can fill up the period found at the end of a sentence (Bone 2018, 22). Asexual, they are neither male nor female, although they can share genetic material through hair-like projections in a process known as conjugation.

While the prokaryote category includes bacteria and archaea, not all bacteria and archaea are prokaryotes. More complex forms are classified as eukaryotes. The tiny archaea prokaryotes thrive in extreme conditions and in this sense are heartier than bacteria. While both of these microbes react to antibiotics, they differ in their response. While many bacteria show susceptibility to a specific antibiotic such as penicillin, archaea may exhibit resistance.

### Prokaryote Cell Structure

Bacteria and archaea cells are about ten times smaller and much more simplified than the cells of eukaryotes. The cellular fluid or cytoplasm that serves as the prokaryotic cell body is surrounded by a cell membrane and usually a cell wall, and sometimes a capsule or slime layer. Inward foldings of the cell membrane called mesosomes are thought to be the site of bacterial respiration.

Prokaryotes have the ability to take up DNA from the environment. Similarly, when a bacterium dies, the cell ruptures and fragments of its DNA spill out and can be taken up by other bacteria. Prokaryotes also share genes with viruses known as bacteriophages, which are their primary predators. Their survival can be enhanced when a bacteriophage transfers DNA from a heartier bacterium.

Because bacteria increase by division, infection can run rampant—for instance, *Escherichia coli* divides every 20 minutes. Some bacteria have a thick layer of material known as glycocalyx located outside their outer cell wall. Glycocalyx is a slimy, gelatinous material produced by the cell membrane, which exists in two forms: a slime layer, which is loosely attached to the cell wall and easily detached; and a capsule, which is a highly organized and firmly attached polysaccharide layer, which may be combined with lipids and proteins. Capsules protect the encapsulated bacteria from being phagocytized (ingested) by phagocytic white blood cells such as the monocytes. Consequently, encapsulated bacteria are able to survive longer in the human body than non-encapsulated bacteria.

Depending on the species, bacteria may have hair-like projections called flagella that aid in movement; thinner hair-like projects known as pili or fimbriae or envelopes that allow bacteria to adhere to surfaces; and thick-walled spores or endospores that are resistant to heat, cold, drying, and most chemicals, allowing certain bacteria to hibernate.

The prokaryotic chromosome usually consists of a single, long, supercoiled, circular DNA molecule. This molecule serves as the control center of the bacterial cell and is capable of duplicating itself, guiding its own cell division, and directing its cellular activities. Prokaryotic cells do not contain nucleoplasm, nor do they contain nuclear membranes. Rather, the chromosome is suspended or embedded in the cytoplasm. Small, circular molecules of double-stranded DNA independent of the chromosome, called plasmids, may also be present in the prokaryotic cells. Plasmids may contain anywhere from fewer than ten genes to several hundred genes (Engelkirk and Duben-Engelkirk 2015, 31).

## Classification of Bacteria

The Domain Bacteria can be divided into kingdoms, phyla, classes, orders, families, genera (plural for genus), and species. The bacterium *Staphylococcus aureus* belongs to the genus *Staphylococcus* and the specific category *aureus*. Together, the words *Staphylococcus aureus* indicate the species.

Bacteria are often named after the infection that they cause. Pneumonia can be caused by *Klebsiella pneumoniae*, *Chlamydophila pneumoniae*, *Streptococcus pneumoniae*, and *Mycoplasma pneumoniae*. Viewed microscopically as a wet preparation from a fecal specimen, bacteria exist as a massive complex of highly motile rods, cocci, diplococci, and oval-shaped yeast buds.

With the use of a Gram stain applied to a bodily fluid dried onto a glass slide, bacteria are classified as gram negative or gram positive depending on the composition of their cell wall and their shape. Bacteria that react with both red and purple stains are called gram variable and further identified with acid-fast stains.

## Archaea

The ancient single-celled microbes in the domain known as Archaea differ from bacteria in that they have different cell wall compositions, as well as different modes of replication, and express genes differently. Bacteria and archaea have different types of ribosomal RNA (rRNA). Archaea have three RNA polymerases like eukaryotes, but bacteria have only one. In addition, archaea have cell walls that lack peptidoglycan and they have membranes that enclose lipids with hydrocarbons rather than the fatty acids found in bacteria.

There are three major known groups of Archaea: methanogens, halophiles (Halobacterium), and thermophiles. The methanogens are anaerobic (i.e., they thrive in oxygen-free environments) microbes that produce methane. The halophiles have a light-sensitive violet pigment called bacteriorhodopsin that provides color and chemical energy. Halophiles can exist in extremely salty water. The thermophiles are classified as such because of their ability to thrive in extreme climates.

## *Eukaryotes*

Although they differ mightily in size and appearance, plants, algae, fungi, and animals are all eukaryotes (Eukarya family) and have similar cell structures. Algae and protozoa are protoists and are classified in the Kingdom Protista. Fungi belong to the Kingdom Fungi, while plants are in the Kingdom Plantae. Animals, including humans, are in the Kingdom Animalia.

Eukaryotes are similar to prokaryotes except that eukaryotes—which can be composed of one cell or many cells (multicellular)—contain a distinct, membrane-bound nucleus. This means that their genetic material, which is present in pairs, is separated from the cytoplasm present in the rest of the cell and is contained in the cell's nucleus.

The large amount of genetic material present in eukaryotic cells means that each cell of an individual organism has a complete copy of all that species' genes. However, all genes are not expressed in every cell. For instance, in animals liver cells express the genes necessary for the liver's appearance and biological functions. Eukaryotic cells specialize by activating a much smaller subset of genes. This arrangement allows animal stem cells to differentiate into different kinds of blood cells depending on the body's needs. Eukaryotic cells also contain mitochondria with their own DNA, which is passed down from the mother, whereas nuclear DNA derived from the cell nucleus is obtained from both parents.

## Eukaryote Cell Structure

The eukaryotic cell is the basic unit of life in numerous microorganisms, plants, and animals, including humans. The eukaryotic cell has its own outer membrane that encloses the cell's contents. This membrane is also called the plasma, cytoplasmic or cellular membrane. Similar to the nuclear membrane surrounding the cell nucleus, the cell membrane selectively regulates the passage of nutrients, waste products, and secretions into and out of the cells. The eukaryotic cell has a nucleus that controls the cell's functions. The nucleus contains a gelatinous matrix or base material known as the nucleoplasm along with chromosomes, as well as a nuclear membrane or outer wall. This membrane contains holes that allow large molecules to enter and exit the nucleus. A semifluid, gelatinous matrix known as cytoplasm or nucleoplasm is distributed between the cell's nucleus and its outer membrane.

## Cytoplasm

The cytoplasm contains insoluble storage granules and various organelles, including the endoplasmic reticulum, ribosomes, Golgi complexes, lysosomes, and centrioles, as well as the mitochondria, the cell's energy factory where most of the adenosine triphosphate molecules are formed by cellular respiration. Defects in the mitochondria of neurons are seen in Alzheimer's disease and described further in Chapter Five.

## Endoplasmic Reticulum

The endoplasmic reticulum is a network of membranous tubules within the cytoplasm of a eukaryotic cell, continuous with the nuclear membrane. It usually has ribosomes attached and is involved in protein and lipid synthesis.

## Ribosomes

Found in both prokaryotic and eukaryotic cells, ribosomes are minute particles consisting of RNA and associated proteins. Ribosomes are distributed in large numbers in the cytoplasm of living cells. Ribosomes bind messenger RNA and transfer RNA to synthesize polypeptides and proteins that govern characteristics such as size. Each eukaryotic ribosome is composed of a large subunit (60S) and a small subunit (40S) that are produced in the cell's nucleolus. The subunits then reside in the cytoplasm, where they release mRNA molecules to initiate protein synthesis. (See also Chapter Twelve.)

## Golgi Complex

The Golgi complex or Golgi apparatus is a stack of flattened, membranous strands that communicates with the endoplasmic reticulum to complete the transformation of newly synthesized proteins into mature, functional ones. These proteins are packaged into small, membrane-enclosed vesicles that can be stored within the cell or exported outside the cell.

## Lysosomes and Peroxisomes

Originating in the Golgi complex, lysosomes are small vesicles that contain lysozyme and other digestive enzymes that break down foreign material that enters the cell through the action of phagocytic cells. If a cell is damaged or worn out, these enzymes help break down the materials, allowing them to be excreted. Peroxisomes are membrane-bound vesicles, which both generate and break down hydrogen peroxide. Peroxisomes contain the enzyme catalase, which assists with the breakdown process. Peroxisomes are especially abundant in the liver cells of mammals.

## Mitochondria and Mitochondrial Dysfunction

Mitochondria, which are reported to have evolved from ancient bacteria (see also the endosymbiotic theory described in Chapter Five), are the power plants of the eukaryotic cell. The thought of humans evolving from the mechanisms used by bacteria to survive may sound strange, but it also explains why the numerous microbes living within and among us have a great influence over our health and wellbeing. In these microscopic organelles known as mitochondria, adenosine triphosphate (ATP) is produced through a process of cellular respiration. Mitochondria also contain their own DNA, which is passed through the matrilineal line from mother to daughter.

Mitochondrial dysfunction, a condition of reduced mitochondrial energy production, has several causes: when there is a loss of maintenance of the electrical and chemical potential of the mitochondria's inner membrane; when alterations in the function of the electron transport chain occur; when there is an inadequate number of mitochondria; or when there is a reduction in the transport of critical metabolites into mitochondria.

Mitochondrial dysfunction occurs in a number of chronic disorders, including neurodegenerative diseases such as Alzheimer's disease, chronic infections, Parkinson's disease, Huntington's disease, amyotrophic lateral sclerosis, and Friedreich's ataxia. Mitochondrial dysfunction is likewise seen in atherosclerosis and other heart and vascular conditions, diabetes, metabolic syndrome, autoimmune diseases, neurobehavioral and psychiatric diseases, autism, chronic fatigue syndrome, Gulf War illnesses, and bipolar disorders, and also as a consequence of aging. Many supplements described in Chapter Twelve, such as alpha lipoic acid, are reported to improve mitochondrial function.

A consequence of the electron transport process involved in the mitochondrial conversion of adenosine diphosphate into adenosine triphosphate is the production of highly reactive free radicals, both reactive oxygen species and reactive nitrogen species. These free radicals can damage cellular lipids, proteins, and DNA, although dismutase enzymes and antioxidants can neutralize this process, providing damage control. However, if the mitochondrial membrane lipids sustain damage, loss of the electrochemical gradient occurs. Damage to the mitochondrial membranes impairs mitochondrial function and causes excess lipid peroxidation (which causes the brown age spots that occur on the skin and in the brain) as a result of excess oxidative stress (Nicolson 2014).

## Cytoskeleton

The cell's cytoskeleton or spine, which is present throughout the cytoplasm, is a system of fibers that provide shape, strength and structure to the cell. The cytoskeletal fibers include microtubules, microfilaments and intermediate filaments.

## Fungi, Protozoa, Plants and Animals

Fungi, protozoa, plants and animals all belong to the *Eukarya* Family. All of these species, like the eukaryotic microorganisms, contain eukaryotic cells with their own genetic material. In their daily interactions with one another, all of the eukaryotes coexist, providing nutrition and sustenance to one another and sometimes harming one another. Both fungi and protozoa have been detected in the brains of individuals with Alzheimer's disease and are discussed further in Chapters Six through Ten.

## Viruses

Viruses are comparatively very small particles called virions that consist of a genome of either DNA or RNA surrounded by a protein coat called a capsid, which is composed of many small protein units called capsomeres. Viruses, which are about eight times smaller than bacteria, are not living cells because they are acellular (i.e., are not made up of cells), and cells are the basic units of life. Viruses appear to be the result of regressive or reverse evolution.

Viewed under a microscope, viruses have an amazing array of shapes, appearing as drums, crystals, chains, bombs and spiders. Viruses are about ten times more numerous than all cells on Earth combined (Bone 2018, 25). More like parasites, they inject the DNA or RNA they have into host cells (hosts can be plants, bacteria, other microbes, and humans), which causes the host cell's machineries to replicate their DNA or RNA and encase the nucleic acid. In doing so, viruses are able to rapidly infect their host. The role of viral infections in AD is described in Chapters Six and Seven.

## The Gut Microbiota and Microbiome

The human gastrointestinal (GI) tract or gut is about 16.5 feet long with a surface area composed of epithelial (tissue) cells and mucus, providing a surface area of approximately 105 feet (Yoo and Mazmanian 2017). Mucin (the basis of mucus) is a type of protein containing an abundance of sugar molecules, resulting in a heavily glycosylated protein. Because of its consistency, mucin forms gels that coat the epithelial linings of organs, including the gastrointestinal track.

Beneath the epithelial layer lies the lamina propria, which is rich in immune system cells, the lumen, and supporting muscles. Blood vessels, neurons and their connections, and glial cells extend through these layers, allowing communication between the gut and the brain. The cells of the GI tract have short life spans and are replaced every two weeks (Strait 2017).

One of the gut's primary functions is to recognize and respond to external changes, such as the presence of pathogens, by communicating this information to the host through an exchange of molecules via the enteric nervous system. The GI tract contains a number of different intestinal epithelial cell (IEC) types with different communication properties. The gut microbes also provide numerous physiological benefits, including strengthening the gut integrity, shaping the intestinal epithelial border, harvesting energy, and regulating host immunity.

About 10–100 trillion microorganisms, from numerous species (including bacteria, archaea, fungi, viruses, protozoa, and spirochetes), are present in the human gut and referred to as the gut microbiota. The term *microbiota* technically refers to the microbial taxa (classes of microbes) associated with humans. The human gut normally contains predominantly bacteria from four phyla—primarily *Firmicutes* and *Bacteroidetes*, with smaller amounts of *Actinobacteria* and *Proteobacteria*, which represent about 98 percent of gut microbes (Hill and Lukiw 2015). The remaining phylotypes are represented by *Cyanobacteria, Fusobacteria, Spirochaetes,* and *Verrucomicrobia*, along with various species of fungi, protozoa and viruses (Gordon et al. 2006).

Researchers describe three different fundamental types of healthy gut microbiomes called enterotypes, each with their own dietary preferences. Each prototype consists of a useful mixture of microbes dominated by *Bacteroides, Prevotella,* or *Ruminococcus*. Individual enterotypes vary depending on ancestral origins, ancient lifestyles and diet. *Bacteroides* prefers to metabolize protein and animal fat; *Prevotella* is linked to mucin proteins and simple carbohydrates; and *Ruminococcus* prefers mucins and sugars (Dietert 2016, 208). In an amended classification, *Ruminococcus* is grouped with *Bacteroides*, resulting in two main enterotypes: *Bacteroides* and *Prevotella*. An abundance of *Bacteroides* has long been associated with colon cancer.

Gut microbes have a number of metabolic functions that are commensal or beneficial to their host and help protect health. Microbes aid in digestion; extract nutrients and energy from food; metabolize xenobiotics; synthesize histamine, amyloid proteins, vitamins B and K, and various neuromodulators such as serotonin; produce several different amino acids and hormones; protect the gut from pathogenic colonization; help neutralize and excrete toxins; and interact with the immune system and the central and peripheral nervous systems.

Perturbations in the gut microbiota affect numerous health conditions. These microbial alterations contribute to disease development and worsen symptoms in type 2 diabetes mellitus, metabolic syndrome, obesity and food cravings, allergies, inflammatory bowel disease, colorectal cancer, multiple sclerosis, neuromyelitis optica spectrum disorders, Parkinson's disease, Huntington's disease, amyotrophic lateral sclerosis and Alzheimer's disease (Ellison 2018).

Alterations in the gut microbiota, particularly a decrease in diversity, can be caused by medications (antibiotics, oral contraceptives, nonsteroidal anti-inflammatory drugs, proton pump inhibitors used for gastric reflux disorders), stress, the ingestion of high amounts of sugar and high-fructose corn syrup, gluten, environmental or food allergies, insomnia, infections, low levels of omega-3 fatty acids and vitamin D, radiation, chemotherapy, extreme exercise, and excessive alcohol (Amen 2017, 99–100).

With rapid changes in antibiotic use, sanitation, and food processing, some of the indigenous microbial species that normally inhabit the gut are at risk for extinction. For the past two decades, researchers have reported that with each new generation, individuals are found to have fewer native microbes. With this loss of diversity, certain conditions are becoming more prominent. For instance, low levels of *Bifidobacterium* and high levels of the fungi *Candida* are related to eczema and allergies (Hyman 2019).

Katherine Harmon writes that the gut microbe *Helicobacter pylori* is facing eradication from heavy antibiotic use. While there are positive outcomes to this development, such as the successful treatment of gastric ulcers and a decrease in gastric cancer, reducing the *Helicobacter pylori* population can increase the risk for various gastric reflux diseases by upsetting the production of hormones and pH levels. In addition, individuals who have *Helicobacter pylori* have been found to have lower risks of childhood asthma, allergic rhinitis, and skin allergies than individuals who do not have *Helicobacter pylori*. This bacterium also mediates the hormone ghrelin, and without it, the altered gut microbiome may contribute to the epidemic of early-life obesity, type 2 diabetes, and metabolic syndrome (Harmon 2009).

The genes of the microbial flora present in the gut are referred to as the gut microbiome, and they account for 99 percent of the genetic material found in the human body. With older methods of identification such as culturing specimens onto aerobic and anaerobic petri dishes, it would be impossible to identify all the different species present in gastrointestinal fluids or fecal specimens. However, with new methods of sequencing micro RNA, the vast array of organisms in the gut can be identified. The microbiome can be evaluated in terms called operational taxonomic units (OTU), with each unit designating a cluster of similar microorganisms.

Approximately 3.3 million genes have been found to make up the human gut microbiome, with new genes added regularly (Qin 2010). For instance, on February 4, 2019, the Wellcome Trust Sanger Institute reported that one hundred new genes were added to the human gut microbiome (Wellcome Trust 2019). To understand the impact of the microbes we coexist with, the human body contains about 22,000 genes. Diversity in the microbiota refers to the measurement of the degree of difference in the microbial species present compared to the species present in the microbiota of one or more other subjects.

Colonization of the gut occurs during birth and is affected by the form of childbirth. A number of studies show that infants born via Caesarean sections (C-sections) lack the protective organisms found in the mother's vaginal canal. Researchers studied the microbiomes of infants born through both C-section and vaginal births using 16S rRNA gene pyrosequencing. The gut microbiomes of infants born via C-section resemble that of the mother's skin, whereas vaginally born infants have microbiomes similar to the vaginal microbiomes of their mothers (Dominguez-Bello 2010). It's thought that the gut's colonization by microbes in early life is a determinant in shaping the colonization of the adult's gut microbiota (Bull and Plummer 2014).

The colonization of the gut with various microorganisms occurs throughout infancy, and at about one to three years of age, the microbiome of children resembles the microbiome of adults. Changes to the gut microbiome in infants are seen with each dietary change—for instance, breastfeeding, introduction of rice, and introduction of formula—and also with the development of fever or the administration of antibiotics. The gut microbiome stays relatively stable throughout life, although personal variations occur, particularly in the elderly (Vogt et al. 2017). The gut's microbiota also receives microbial additions via secretions from the oral and nasal cavities.

A healthy gut microbiome has lots of diversity. However, herbicides and antibiotics can destroy normal flora, leaving an abundance of bacterial strains, fungi, and parasites that are resistant to antibiotics. Researchers at Washington University Medical School have found that mice treated with antibiotics developed a significant reduction in killer T lymphocytes (killer T cells), which are essential for initiating the immune response. As a consequence, these mice were resistant to attack by viruses and developed severe viral disease (Bhandari 2018).

With a reduction in diversity, the microbiome may no longer be able to manage its usual health-promoting functions and produce the appropriate types and amounts of hormones, vitamins, and neurotransmitters. Other factors that can cause changes to the gut microbiome include dietary changes (especially during travel to a foreign country rife with different endemic microorganisms); lack of dietary fiber; deficiencies in vitamins, minerals and other nutrients; malabsorption syndromes; various medicines; and introduction of new microorganisms through poor oral hygiene or contaminated food sources.

## Microbiome-Produced Amyloids

Many different microbiome species, including bacteria and fungi, are known to secrete amyloid proteins. The extracellular amyloids known as curli fibers, composed of major structural subunit CsgA, are produced by *Escherichia coli*. Biofilms are found to consist of amyloids, microbes and lipoproteins. The extracellular CsgA amyloid precursor protein contains a pathogen-associated molecular pattern that is recognized by the immune system's toll-like receptor 2 (TLR2), similar to its recognition of amyloid beta (Aβ) 42 (Hill and Lukiw 2015). The ability of many microbes to produce vast amounts of amyloids indicates that humans are exposed to a large amyloid burden, which is especially pronounced in aged individuals whose blood-brain barrier and gastrointestinal lining are more permeable.

## The Gut Microbiota in Alzheimer's Disease

The gut microbiota in people with AD is significantly different from the gut microbiota of sex-matched control subjects without dementia. Overall, in AD there is less diversity, with fewer species of microbes than typically seen. There are also significantly fewer *Firmicutes, Actinobacteria,* and *Bifidobac-*

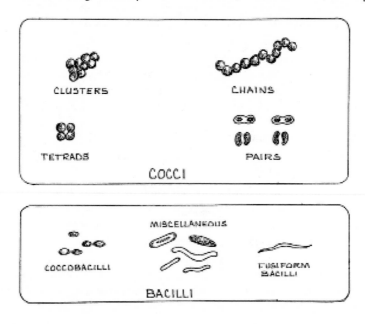

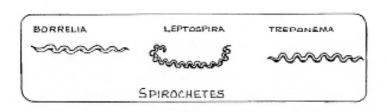

**Cellular Morphologies of Bacteria.**

*terium* species in the microbiome of AD patients and marked increases in *Bacteriodetes* species.

*Firmicutes* is normally the main bacterial phylum, comprising more than 250 distinct genera, including *Lactobacillus, Streptococcus, Mycoplasma,* and *Clostridium,* microbes that produce several short-chain fatty acids (SCFAs) such as butyrate. In the intestines, butyrate regulates fluid transport, ameliorates mucosal inflammation and oxidative status, reinforces the epithelial lining, and modulates visceral sensitivity and intestinal motility. A growing number of studies has indicated that adequate butyrate is needed to prevent colon cancer.

In one study of the gut microbiome in AD, Nicholas Vogt and his colleagues at the University of Wisconsin examined the microbiome as well as the cerebrospinal fluid (CSF) markers of patients who also had CSF specimens obtained for a different study. They found that the markers of AD in the CSF of subjects whose gut microbiome suggested AD were also elevated. The markers of AD studied in the spinal fluid samples included tests for Aβ-40, Aβ-42 and tau protein (Vogt et al. 2017).

With less diversity in the microbiota of AD patients, the lipopolysaccharides and amyloids released by the bacterium *Escherichia coli* and other microbes become more abundant. The increased production of amyloid proteins in the gut may trigger increased amyloid production in the brain. Lipopolysaccharides released from gram-negative bacterial cell membranes can also travel to the brain and injure neurons. Immune system changes caused by the curli proteins secreted by *Escherichia coli* trigger alterations in the immune system, including increased expression of TLR2, interleukin-6 (IL-6), and tumor necrosis factor. Increased levels of these immune system chemical cytokines are found in patients with AD (Kowalski and Mulak 2019).

The microbiome in AD patients is associated with dysregulation of the anti-inflammatory P-glycoprotein pathway. The microbiota-gut-brain is a bidirectional communication system. In one study, researchers examined stool specimens from 108 nursing home residents for five months, studying T84 intestinal epithelial function for P-glycoprotein (P-gp) expression. P-gp is a critical mediator of intestinal homeostasis (cells and bodily systems working together to maintain health).

Besides clinical parameters, the researchers found numerous microbial taxa and intact genes that can be used as predictors of AD when compared to elders in the study with good cognitive function. In vitro studies using the stools from AD patients and incorporating aliquots of these stool samples into stool samples taken from patients without dementia lowered P-gp expression levels, confirming decreased microbial homeostasis in AD patients (Haran et al. 2019).

Lipopolysaccharides (endotoxins shed from the membranes of gram-negative bacteria) are able to produce amyloid proteins. Blood levels of these polysaccharides in AD patients are 3 times the level seen in age-matched controls (Zhan et al. 2018). Markers of inflammation such as C-reactive protein and IL-6 have been found to be elevated in the blood of AD patients several years before overt symptoms of dementia emerge.

Experimental studies also show that injections of bacterial lipopolysaccharides into the fourth ventricle of the brain cause many of the same pathological and inflammatory changes seen in the brains of AD patients (Kowalski and Mulak 2019). While signals transmitted from the gut can travel through the vagus nerve to the brain, many of the gut microbes and their products that migrate to the brain are a result of leaky gut syndrome and defects in the blood-brain barrier.

## The Gut Microbiome's Influence on Blood Lipids

Because of the gut microbiome's involvement with cardiovascular disease, researchers investigated the role of the gut microbiome on blood lipid variations and body mass index (BMI). Higher microbial diversity was correlated with a lower BMI and lower triglyceride levels and a higher level of high-density lipoprotein (HDL—the "good" cholesterol) (Fu et al. 2015). The link between elevated cholesterol and AD has long been established. However, recent studies show that other lipid families (such as phospholipids) play a role in the synaptic dysfunction and loss of communication between neurons in AD (Di Paola and Kim 2011).

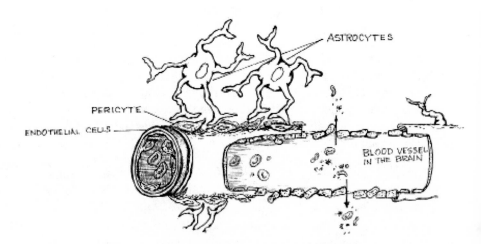

Diseased Blood-Brain Barrier (BBB).

## Dysregulation of Inflammatory Pathways in the AD Gut Microbiome

The bidirectional communication system between the gut microbiota and the brain has been poorly understood in AD, although the association with bacterial infections and inflammation-related immunosenescence has long been known. Recent studies show that stool samples from elderly AD subjects can lead to lower P-glycoprotein expression levels compared to samples from age-matched subjects without dementia. This loss of dysregulation seen in AD subjects is thought to be responsible for the low levels of butyrate seen and the higher abundance of bacterial taxa known to cause pro-inflammatory states (Haran et al. 2019).

## Gut Dysbiosis

Imbalances and alterations in the gut microbiota and its host result in a condition of gut dysbiosis. Animal studies using mice show that dietary changes, especially high-fat diets, can cause significant changes in bacterial metabolism (particularly in the production of short-chain fatty acids and amino acids) in as little as one week and can lead to large changes after only one day (Ursell 2012).

Dysbiosis of the microbiota along with infections from viruses are responsible for a number of diseases, including chronic infection, liver disease, metabolic diseases, gastrointestinal cancer, pulmonary diseases, and autoimmune diseases, as well as mental and psychological disorders (Sochocka et al. 2017). Metabolic changes caused by dysbiosis include changes to lipids and bile acids, which are described later in this chapter. Moreover, imbalances in the gut microbiota can result in inflammation that is associated with the pathogenesis of obesity, type 2 diabetes mellitus, and AD.

Dysbiosis attributed to the use of antibiotics usually resolves within a week of stopping the antibiotic. However, with the use of more modern broad-spectrum antibiotics such as ciprofloxacin, the changes in the gut microbiota persist longer and include a decrease in the richness, diversity and evenness of the remaining microflora. Some species are slow to return, taking as long as four years before the normal gut flora is reestablished. The use of dietary interventions, prebiotics and probiotics to help restore microbial balance to the gut is described in Chapter Twelve.

When it comes to healing from dysbiosis, the gut microbiota appears to be more plastic than originally thought. With appropriate dietary measures and the judicious use of probiotics, dysbiosis can be reversed. A hint that there is greater plasticity in this regard than previously thought is the ability to successfully treat *Clostridium difficile* infection and autoimmune disease patients, particularly those with multiple sclerosis, with fecal transplant treatments. Despite this plasticity, the gut microbiomes in patients with Alzheimer's disease exhibit significant persistent perturbations.

## Enteric Nervous System

The enteric network consists of the gut's nervous, endocrine, and immune systems. Embedded within its epithelial layer, the gut's surface area contains 70–80 percent of the body's immune system cells, more than one million neurons, and up to 100,000 extrinsic nerve endings (Yoo and Mazmanian 2017). Precise interactions between the nervous and immune systems of the gut allow the gut to respond to dietary products, foreign antigens, medications, invasive pathogenic microbes, and the gut's own diverse microbiota.

The enteric nervous system is well aware of changes and threats to the

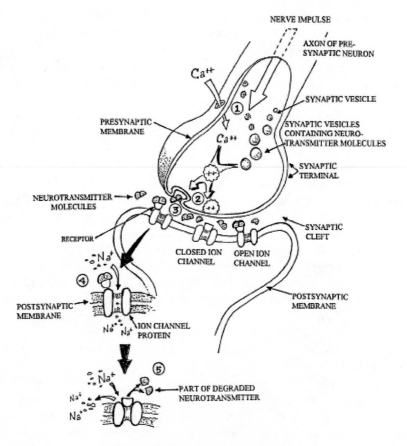

**Transmission of Nerve Impulses.**

gastrointestinal system and reacts by translating external chemical signals into neuronal impulses that are transmitted to other organs throughout the body, including the central nervous system. Known as the mind-body connection, the nervous system, endocrine system, and immune system influence one another in an effort to maintain homeostasis. The vagus and pelvic nerves efficiently send signals from the gut to the brain.

The enteric nervous system is an additional site for amyloid precursor protein (APP) and its processing, which results in the production of amyloid proteins and oligomers. The presence of APP in the enteric nervous system is more evidence of its role in the pathogenesis of AD.

## Enteric Endocrine System

The gastrointestinal tract is the largest endocrine organ in the body. The endocrine cells residing there, scattered among the epithelial cells, are referred to as the enteric endocrine system. Enteric endocrine cells react to changes in the gut and help control digestion by secreting the hormones gastrin, cholecystokinin, and secretin. Hormones produced in other endocrine glands, such as the pancreas, also communicate with the nervous system and secrete hormones as needed. Neuropeptides are small protein molecules capable of cell communication that are produced by neuroendocrine cells, which receive signals from neurons and respond by secreting endocrine hormones or neuropeptides.

The hypothalamic-pituitary-adrenal axis, or HPA axis, is another mechanism by which the brain communicates with the gut to help control digestion through the action of hormones. The enteric nervous system, through its ability to affect gut transit time and the secretion of mucus by the gut's epithelial cells, can help dictate which microbes inhabit the gut.

Cellular communication can also be disrupted by the gut's microbiota. Bacterial residents of the gut, especially gram-negative microorganisms, can secrete large amounts of amyloids and lipopolysaccharides, which can damage neurons and interfere with communication between the signaling pathways.

## *The Brain-Gut-Microbiota Axis and Epigenetics*

In recent years, researchers have found that the brain and gut are able to communicate with one another through a network of neural, immune, cytokine (immune system chemicals), endocrine and metabolic pathways. This bidirectional communication occurs between the microbes in the gut and neurons via chemicals and hormones that constantly provide feedback regarding feelings of hunger, stress, illness, or ingestion of a toxin. Known as the brain-gut-microbiota axis, this feedback system can cause a feeling of butterflies in one's stomach during conditions of nervousness or anxiety.

Often referred to as the second brain, the gut can send its own relaxation-inducing neurotransmitters such as serotonin back to the brain. Most of the body's serotonin is produced in the gut. The gut's resident microbes also produce essential nutrients such as vitamin K, which plays an important role in blood coagulation. In addition, microbes residing in the gut produce a range of neuroactive chemicals, including kynurenine, melatonin, catecholamines, histamine, acetylcholine, and gamma-aminobutyric acid. Commensal gut microbes also metabolize the amino acid tryptophan. Dysregulation of tryptophan's metabolite, serotonin, is a characteristic finding in patients with AD (Sochocka et al. 2018).

Other metabolites produced by bacteria may also interfere with brain function and, to varying degrees, damage the blood-brain barrier, allowing substances to move freely from the gut to the brain. Short-chain fatty acids, particularly butyrate (butyric acid), acetate, and propionate, can modulate signals sent to the peripheral and central nervous systems. In addition, butyrate can damage cholinergic neurons in the gut, increasing gut motility. However, butyrate also has a neuroprotective effect on the brain. In mice, butyrate improved contextual memory, even in those in the late stages of AD (Dietert 2016, 191; Sochocka et al. 2018).

Bile acids are primarily metabolized in the liver with contributions from gut microbes. Studies show that gut microbiome–produced bile acids are increased in individuals with AD and are associated with functional and structural brain changes, including cognitive decline, reduced brain glucose metabolism, and greater brain atrophy, as well as increased accumulations of amyloid and tau proteins (Alzheimer's Association 2018).

## Epigenetics

Humans are reported to have approximately 22,000 genes. However, not all genes are turned on or expressed. An underwhelming number of these genes, by themselves, cannot sustain human life. For this reason, humanity's second genome, provided courtesy of the microbiome, is necessary because it has the ability to switch on human genes or switch these genes off. For instance, the production of embryonic rather than adult hemoglobin in a human fetus is under the control of these epigenetic gene switches. Specifically, hemoglobin production in the embryo is under the control of sodium butyrate produced by gut microbes.

Epigenetics refers to ways in which proteins are expressed through molecular processes that differ from the instructions in the DNA sequence.

These processes can be triggered by one's experiences and environment, including diet. A common example is DNA methylation. Here, a methyl group (CH3) binds to the nucleotides of the DNA itself and controls how often that gene is expressed (Heine 2017, 28). DNA methylation is explained further in Chapter Eleven.

In *The Human Superorganism*, Rodney Dietert explains that complex biological functions (including the formation and maintenance of memories, the effectiveness of the immune response, the quality of sperm production, and the levels of various hormones) are all under a certain level of epigenetic control. In addition, these switches, which have their own memory of past generations, can be programmed and influenced by gut microbes so that certain genes are switched on at different times during development (Dietert 2016, 87).

## Bacterial Amyloids and Curli Fibrils

The gut microbiota is a significant source of bacterial amyloid protein. The most studied gut amyloid is the curli fibril produced by *Escherichia coli*. Amyloids are sticky proteins that help bacterial cells to hold together in forming biofilms and to resist destruction by physical or immune factors. Bacterial amyloids differ from the central nervous system amyloids in their primary structure, but similarities in their tertiary structure exist to a degree that could cause their presence to stimulate an immune response and the production of neuronal amyloid in the brain. Researchers have found that the presence of curli proteins in the brain caused increased expression of pro-inflammatory cytokines. In a process of molecular mimicry, bacterial amyloids may act as prion-like proteins, in which one amyloidogenic protein (curli, tau, amyloid beta protein, alpha-syn and prion) causes another to form the beta-sheet structure of misfolded protein seen in AD (Kowalski and Mulak 2019).

# *Alterations Along the Gut-Liver-Brain Axis in AD*

At the 2018 Alzheimer's Association International Conference, researchers described an association with the liver, gut, and brain. Specifically, as other studies have noted, the brain in AD has low levels of plasmalogens, lipid molecules essential for cell membranes (Alzheimer's Association 2018; Mushegian 2018).

Plasmalogens are phospholipid molecules defined by the presence of an alkene group next to a vinyl ether linkage. Having evolved in the early days of life on earth, plasmalogens are found in animals and many different anaerobic bacteria (Goldfine 2018). The plasmalogen lipids include the omega-3 fatty acids docosahexaenoic acid (DHA) and eicosapentaenoic acid (EPA), the omega-6 fatty acid adrenic acid and closely related lipids. In humans, plasmalogens produced in the liver are abundant in the heart and brain, where they're used to make cell membranes and mediate signals. Plasmalogens are reported to be 60 percent lower in the brain cell membranes of individuals with AD compared to normal subjects (Mushegian 2018).

Fragile molecules, plasmalogens are susceptible to light, have poor solubility and possess limited lifespans, which has made studying them difficult. But, facing the question of why plasminogen levels were diminished in AD, researchers at George Washington University set out to find the reason. They discovered that the mitochondrial enzyme, cytochrome c, along with another lipid catalyzes the oxidative cleavage of the vinyl ether bond, destroying the plasmalogen molecule. To summarize, mitochondrial dysfunction releases cytochrome c, and in conditions of oxidative stress, the bonds that hold plasmalogen molecules together are broken. The chemical reaction results in increased production of alpha-hydroxyaldehyde, a chemical found at high concentrations in the brains of patients with AD that is associated with disease severity. The role of reactive chlorine species in plasmalogen breakdown during the immune response is described in Chapter Four.

Researchers at the 18th Alzheimer's Association International Conference described a study measuring the ratios of fifteen bile acid metabolites in individuals identified by neuroimaging tests as having early-stage AD or who were at high risk for AD. Bile salts are synthesized from cholesterol in the liver, and bacteria in the gut also produce them. Bile salts have hormonal actions throughout the body and function to allow digestion of dietary fats, oils and cholesterol.

Supported by a grant from the National Institutes of Health–led Accelerating Medicines Partnership–Alzheimer's Disease (AMP-AD) program, the researchers compared the bile salt findings with levels of amyloid beta (Aβ) and tau protein in cerebrospinal fluid (CSF). They found increased levels of bile acids produced by gut bacteria in the brains of individuals with AD. These increases were associated with functional and structural brain changes, including cognitive decline, reduced brain glucose metabolism, and greater brain atrophy. These bile acids were also associated with increased amyloid and tau accumulations in CSF (Alzheimer's Association 2018).

Researchers from the Erasmus Medical Center in Rotterdam also described genetic variants, particularly APOE-ε4 and SORL1, which were associated with decreased levels in some lipids involved in the health and repair of brain cell membranes. In addition, the researchers reported that bile acids cluster with caffeine molecules in the blood, which might suggest a possibility for lifestyle interventions.

Researchers in the ADMC and UC Davis–West Coast Metabolomics Center reported on their studies of 400 different lipids in AD at the 18th International AD Conference. Their subjects from the AD Neuroimaging Initiative included 200 dementia-free individuals, 400 subjects with mild cognitive impairment and 200 subjects with AD. Using a new method designed to cluster lipids by chemical similarity, they correlated lipid levels in AD subjects with the degree of brain atrophy, their amyloid and tau levels, and severity of cognitive decline.

These researchers concluded that lipid metabolism is disturbed in AD patients. Specific deficits were seen in proper incorporation of unsaturated fatty acids, primarily the omega-3 lipids EPA and DHA, and arachidonic acid. Obese and male subjects showed the most marked disturbances (Alzheimer's Association 2018). While the addition of fish oil has not proved beneficial in clinical trials, new studies are under way using other lipid supplements. Treatments addressing liver function are another possibility.

## Leaky Gut Syndrome

Leaky gut syndrome is a condition in which the tight junctions of the gut's outer membrane become damaged, allowing for the inadvertent release of potentially harmful substances like microorganisms, toxins and undigested food particles to enter the bloodstream. Dysbiosis of the gut can cause this increase in intestinal permeability. Other factors reported to cause leaky gut syndrome include glyphosate in RoundUp and non-steroidal anti-inflammatory drugs such as ibuprofen, alcohol, and medicines for constipation, particularly MiraLAX (Bush 2019), as well as protein pump inhibitors and oral contraceptives.

The immune system, in responding to these antigenic particles, launches a response that can lead to the development of many different autoimmune and neurodegenerative conditions. Dementia is associated with the production of inflammatory cytokines—for instance, IL-beta, which reduces the normal phagocytosis (ingestion by phagocyte white blood cells) of amyloid beta and leads to NLRP3-inflammasome activation, which causes the release of cytokines such as caspase-1 and IL-18, which lead to increased production of amyloid beta deposits.

Common symptoms of leaky gut syndrome include mental fog, diarrhea, immune system dysfunction, headaches, sugar cravings, joint pain, and excessive fatigue. A fecal test for gut dysbiosis can be used to help diagnose leaky gut syndrome. Therapeutic dietary interventions with an emphasis on omega-3 fatty acids are described in Chapter Twelve.

## Summary

This chapter provides an overview of the microbial world from its earliest origins to its necessary presence in the human body. The basic microbial classes and their cell structures are described to introduce the reader to the cellular interactions that humans and microbes share and rely on.

The microflora of the normal gut and their biochemical functions are described and compared to the changes in the gut microbiota that are seen in patients with AD. Disruptions of the gut microflora result in conditions of dysbiosis. Dysbiosis disrupts numerous intricate metabolic functions. These changes, along with alterations in the gut's outer layer, result in biochemical changes in the brains of individuals with Alzheimer's disease and a response by the immune system that leads to neuroinflammation and neurodegeneration.

Alterations to lipopolysaccharides, short-chain free fatty acids, lipids and bile salts in AD offer supporting evidence regarding the role that infections and dysbiosis play in disrupting cell signaling and evoking pro-inflammatory-directed immune changes that contribute to the development of AD.

# FOUR

# The Immune System, Neurodegeneration and the Blood-Brain Barrier

This chapter serves as an introduction to the immune system and the response that it launches when the body is injured or attacked by pathogenic microbes. Inflammation is one of the immune system's first lines of protective defense, and when it targets the cells of the brain, it causes a condition of neuroinflammation, which, over time, can injure neurons, causing neurodegenerative disease. While the blood-brain barrier functions to shield the brain from toxins and bacteria, disruptions in this barrier allow for the entry of pathogens and toxic chemicals that interfere with normal signaling. Dysbiosis and other disruptions to the gut microbiome, infections, and reactivation of latent viruses can all initiate an immune response that leads to inflammation in the brain (neuroinflammation) and neurodegenerative diseases, including Alzheimer's disease.

In chronic infection, changes to immune cells and the many chemicals they produce are commonly seen. The brains of patients with AD show evidence of these changes, including changes in T lymphocytes, complement and activated microglial cells.

## Immune System Network

The immune system is an intricate network of organs, cells, and chemical molecules with complex pathways working together to defend the body. Having the power of selective discrimination, immune system cells are able to distinguish an individual's own cells and tissues (self) from foreign protein molecules.

The immune system functions to protect the body from foreign sub-

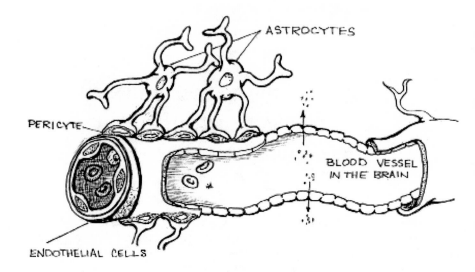

**Healthy Blood-Brain Barrier (BBB).**

stances, such as toxins, pollen, protein, lipid, and carbohydrate molecules present in microorganisms; to launch an immune response against pathogens and foreign antigens that have entered the body; to stop the growth of neoplastic, damaged or infected tissue cells; and to initiate a specific line of defense (for instance, the production of antibodies to destroy invading substances).

The immune system consists of (1) primary lymphoid organs, such as the bone marrow and thymus, the major sites of white blood cell production; (2) secondary lymphoid tissue, including the spleen, appendix, tonsils, adenoids, lymph nodes, lymph fluid, skin, and discrete clusters of immune system cells that line the urogenital and gastrointestinal tracts; (3) immune system cells, primarily lymphocytes, macrophages, and dendritic cells; and (4) potent chemicals such as the cytokines and complement, which are able to modulate the immune response.

The bone marrow is akin to a central repository. It is responsible for producing and storing white blood cells and sending them out into the blood circulation or to other immune system organs as needed. Certain white blood cells known as T lymphocytes are sent to the thymus gland to mature. The thymus is an endocrine gland situated below the thyroid. Here, immature T lymphocytes destined to become autoreactive (and contribute to autoimmune disease development) are either eliminated or rendered inert. Healthy T lymphocytes mature and learn their functions of recognizing and tolerating self-antigens and distinguishing self from the foreign protein antigens they need to defend against. Other cells, including non-specialized lymphocytes, epithelial cells, and macrophages, also mature in the thymus gland.

The secondary lymphoid tissue receives white blood cells from the primary lymphoid tissues and stores them until they are needed. The immune system works in conjunction with the lymphatic system to release both T and B lymphocyte cells from lymph nodes to help in launching an immune response. Areas of lymphoid tissue are also concentrated in the gastrointestinal tract, the respiratory tract, and the urogenital tract.

Stem cells produced in the bone marrow, sternum, skull, hips, ribs and spine are immature precursor cells that can differentiate into specific tissue cells as needed. Stem cells are also found in the blood supplying the umbilical cord (cord blood) and are rarely present in the peripheral blood circulation.

## The Innate and Adaptive Immune Systems

The immune system has two primary lines of defense: the innate immune system and the adaptive immune system. The innate immune system is a natural mechanism that distinguishes self from foreign (not natural to the body) non-specific protein antigens such as viruses, bacteria and pollen or the proteins that these antigens release. Present at birth in a rudimentary form, the innate immune system doesn't fully emerge until humans reach one to two years of age. The innate immune system consists of (1) barriers, such as skin; (2) secretions such as tears or mucus to help move infection away from vital organs; and (3) a generalized immune response orchestrated by white blood cells that creates a number of effects, including inflammation, a cascade of complement proteins, and non-specific cellular responses.

Antibodies produced by an innate immune system reaction generally last for the individual's lifetime. For instance, someone infected with the rubella virus develops measles (also known as German measles) and has lifelong antibodies that grant immunity from developing measles again. Blood tests for rubella antibodies can also be used to confirm that an individual had measles in the past. While the innate immune system responds quickly, it lacks a memory to identify subsequent pathogenic attacks.

The adaptive or acquired immune system is more complex and develops as specific foreign proteins begin to attack the body, such as cytomegalovirus rather than all viruses. The adaptive immune system employs specialized cells (particularly T and B lymphocyte cells) that lead to the production of antibodies against specific microorganisms, such as the Epstein-Barr virus. The production of protective antibodies in one's own body is called active acquired immunity and is usually long lasting, whereas in passive acquired immunity the individual receives antibodies produced by other people or (in some cases) animals. This type of immunity is usually temporary. An example would be antibodies passively transferred through the placental membrane to infants.

Vaccines cause conditions of artificial active acquired immunity. Vaccines contain treated preparations of infectious agents that render them inert. When someone is vaccinated, their immune system reacts as if they were exposed to the infectious agent. This reaction causes the immune system to produce specific antibodies against the infectious agent, conferring immunity.

## Humoral and Cell-Mediated Immunity

The immune system has two major arms that drive the immune response. Humoral (also called antibody-mediated) immunity occurs when the immune system produces antibodies against a specific protein antigen (infectious microorganism). These protective antibodies are effective in destroying the antigen when it is encountered again. Cell-mediated immunity (CMI) involves a complex interaction among many white blood cells and the chemical cytokines that these cells produce. The white blood cells involved in CMI include macrophages, T helper (Th) and T cytotoxic (Tc) lymphocytes, natural killer (NK) cells and granulocytic segmented neutrophils. In CMI, a macrophage first engulfs and then partially digests a pathogenic microbe, initiating a cascade of steps in which the pathogen is destroyed. In CMI, antibodies are rarely involved, appearing only if a simultaneous humoral immune response occurs.

## The Neuroimmune System Cells

The neuroimmune system is a finely tuned network composed of glial cells and signaling molecules that reside in the central nervous system and the immune system. The neuroimmune system mobilizes host defenses against infectious microbes and other pathogens and helps to heal and remove damaged neurons.

Ninety percent of the cells in the human brain are glial cells (Kabba et al. 2018). The primary glial cells include macroglia (astrocytes, oligodendrocytes) and microglia. Glial cells function to support neurons and provide the brain with structure. They also separate and occasionally insulate neuronal groups and synaptic connections. In addition, glial cells have housekeeping chores such as removing debris after injury or neuronal death and ensuring efficient signaling between neurons. At the junctions with nerve-muscle cell synapses, glial cells regulate the properties of the presynaptic terminal.

Astrocytes, which are the most abundant of the glial cells, help create an impermeable lining in the brain's capillaries and venules. Known as the blood-brain barrier (BBB), this lining prevents toxic substances from entering the brain. Astrocytes help to maintain the appropriate potassium ion concentration in the extracellular space between neurons needed for the nerve cell's firing of signals.

Star shaped astrocytes have rather long processes that may be employed in nurturing distant cells. Astrocytes that place end-feet on the brain's blood vessels cause the vessels' interior endothelial lining to form the tight junctions of the BBB. (Disruptions to the BBB are described in Chapter Five.) Other glial cells are thought to release growth factors and help nourish neurons (Kandel et al. 2000, 20).

Microglia, which are considered resident phagocytes (able to engulf and destroy other cells) in the brain, are derived from macrophages in the myeloid cell line (having a progenitor cell that makes granulocytes, red blood cells and platelets). Microglia stay in constant communication with the brain's other cells and regulate homeostasis by facilitating migration of mature neurons, modulating synaptic functions and pruning excessive synaptic growth in developing neurons. Microglia also regulate the extracellular microenvironment by buffering water concentrations, insulating axons and helping maintain the permeability of the blood-brain barrier.

When glial cells perceive that there is a threat, such as the presence of a pathogen in the nervous system, the cells become activated. Upon activation, the cells release cytokines and chemokines and launch a major immune response characterized by neuroinflammation.

The specific immune response launched (including the types of cytokines released) depends on the disease threat and disease process. Different inflammatory markers are seen in different conditions. Microglia and macrophages react the same to assaults from the central nervous system and the peripheral system. Macrophages in peripheral tissues and microglia in the brain launch the first line of defense for the innate immune system. Microglia can be primed toward the M1 (pro-inflammatory) mode by stimulation with lipopolysaccharides released from bacteria or by interferon-gamma. Macrophages can also be activated to express the M2 anti-inflammatory phenotype by parasitic products or associated signals projecting resolution and repair.

## Immune System Cells

White blood cells (leukocytes) are the most important immune system cells. Leukocytes that launch an innate immune response include granulocytic neutrophils, lymphocytes, monocytes, dendrites, macrophages, cytotoxic natural killer (NK) cells and some early progenitor cells such as myelocytes.

In the adaptive immune system, the major players are lymphocytes, particularly the subsets known as T and B lymphocytes (T and B cells). While mast cells—basophilic granulocytes primarily found in connective tissue—are not normally present in the blood circulation, they are quick to join in the innate immune response. When mast cells are activated, they release cytokines and cellular granules that contain chemical molecules that initiate an inflammatory cascade described later in this chapter. Mast cells also release chemical mediators, such as histamine. Histamine causes blood vessels to dilate, facilitating movement of immune cells and chemicals to areas of the body where they are most needed.

Dendritic cells (dendrites) are antigen-presenting cells that help T lymphocytes alert B lymphocytes to respond. Dendrites are located in tissues and can move to external environments in the skin and eyes and also the inner mucosal lining of the nasopharyngeal system, stomach, and intestines. Since dendritic cells are located in tissues that are the usual sites for initial infection, they can identify foreign threats and alert other immune system cells. Dendritic cells function in both the innate immune system and the adaptive immune system.

## T and B Lymphocytes

During their process of maturation in the thymus gland, T lymphocytes are programmed by virtue of T receptors on their surface membranes to react only with specific antigens, such as protein particles from specific viruses or parasites. Since the immune system is capable of reacting with thousands of different antigens, there are only a few cells of each type in residence at any given time. However, T cells have the ability to multiply and produce identical clones as needed to respond to an attack by specific antigens, particularly pathogenic microorganisms.

Because they have available immunoglobulin protein for antibody production on their cell membranes, B lymphocytes are able to produce antibodies to help fight against infectious microorganisms or allergens. B cells function in the adaptive immune system and only make antibodies when they receive the appropriate command signal from T cells. T cells act as scouts, always vigilantly guarding the body against threats and alerting B cells when the need arises.

Upon recognizing a foreign antigen, T cells release a specific chemical called a cytokine that functions to alert B cells. In an intricately orchestrated process, the B cell is able to (1) differentiate into an immunoglobulin-rich plasma cell capable of producing antibodies that target specific protein antigens or (2) become a memory B lymphocyte that stores information and produces these particular antibodies at another time.

## Subsets of T Lymphocytes

When laboratories first created methods to differentiate T lymphocytes in subclasses, the two main types of T lymphocytes were the helper cells and suppressor cells. Following the development of more sophisticated methods of classifying T cells, more subtypes have been identified. The main subtypes of T cells now include:

- Suppressor or regulatory cells (Treg cells), which regulate the immune response by suppressing pathogenic, autoreactive, and neoplastic cells (anti-inflammatory effect)
- Gamma delta T cells, which are tissue-specific cells that are rapidly activated during infection
- Cytotoxic T cells (Tc cells, CD8+ cells), which destroy virally infected host cells, pathogenic cells and tumor cells
- Mucosal-associated invariant T cells (MAITs), which activate other cells to respond to pathogens
- Memory T cells, which are long-lived T cells that have previously encountered the microorganism or neoplastic cell and are able to react quickly and with greater intensity
- Effector T cells, which include activated helper and cytotoxic T cells involved in the immune response to infectious and neoplastic antigens
- Helper T cells (CD4+ cells), which are especially important in the innate immune response, where they help by releasing cytokines, which modulate the immune response

## Th1 and Th2 CD4+ Helper Cells

Depending on the cytokines available, T helper lymphocytes can develop into Th1 or Th2 cells. Normally, individuals have about the same amount of each cell type. Th1 cells promote cellular immunity, encourage inflammation, and have anti-cancer and antiviral properties. Th1 cytokines such as interleukin-2 (IL-2) and interferon-gamma (IFN-gamma) dominate in organ-specific autoimmune diseases when low levels of Th2 cells fail to halt overproduction of Th1 cells.

Th2 cells have an anti-inflammatory effect and work to control the process of inflammation to prevent persistent inflammation. Th2 cells promote humoral immunity and are more often associated with normal immune responses such as mild allergic reactions and asthma. Th2 cytokines such as the interleukins IL-4, IL-5, and IL-10 are commonly seen in autoimmune disorders. An increased number of activated TCD4+ cells is seen in the peripheral blood of patients with AD along with increases in IL-17, IL-6, IL-1 and TNF-alpha compared to normal control subjects (Pirker-Kees et al. 2013; Oberstein et al. 2018).

Th17 effector cells, a subset of the CD4+ lineage, are induced in parallel with Th1 cells when a pro-inflammatory response is required. A collaborative potential between Th1 and Th17 cells results in directing neutrophils to the microorganisms or cells targeted by the response. Th17 cells produce a variety of IL-17 cytokines (ILA-ILE). IL-17 has also been shown to play a role in the production of matrix metalloproteinase, an enzyme that functions to degrade tissue during an inflammatory response. While IL-17 collaborates with Th1, in the presence of other cytokines such as IFN-gamma, IL-17 can have an antagonistic effect (Damsker et al. 2010).

## Immune Cells of the Gastrointestinal Systems

The gastrointestinal tract houses the main portion of the immune system. Rich in cells and chemical molecules of the innate and adaptive immune systems, the immune responses originating in the gastrointestinal tract are aided by molecules from the enteric nervous and endocrine systems. Pathogenic microorganisms and toxins regularly enter the body through food sources, medications, saliva and secretions from the oral and nasal cavities. The enteric immune cells are on continual alert to tolerate the beneficial nutrient-rich protein antigens and launch an attack against the pathogenic molecules.

The immune system cells are aided in these tasks by having a highly efficient mucosal barrier interfaced with the gut's epithelial lining along with a highly specialized enteric immune system composed of a large population of scattered immune cells mainly located on Peyer's patches in the organized mucosal lymphoid tissues termed the gut-associated lymphoid tissue (GALT). Antigens enter the gastric mucosa through microfold cells (M cells), which then transport the antigens to the GALT area for further processing and an adaptive immune response if needed. Enteric glial cells also contribute to a healthy GALT by virtue of their surface's toll-like receptors and ability to release signaling molecules.

In an animal study conducted on mice, researchers found that the presence of the anaerobic gram-positive segmented filamentous bacteria *Arthromitus* in the gut resulted in TH17 cell differentiation on CD4+ T cells and increased production of IL-17 (Ivanov et al. 2019).

## Complement

The complement system includes a large army of proteins that become activated in the presence of pathogens. Complement proteins are located throughout the body, with high concentrations in the gastrointestinal tract and low concentrations in the brain. In a series of steps known as a cascade (which has three different pathways), complement proteins interact to opsonize bacteria (i.e., make bacteria more susceptible to engulfment), recruit phagocytes with complement receptors to engulf the bacterial Aβ, and destroy certain bacteria by creating a membrane-attack-complex (MAC) that causes the formation of pores in the bacterial membranes. Because complement is heat-labile, it augments the opsonization of bacteria by specific antibodies that target specific bacteria and allows these antibodies to kill some bacteria. In this way, complement protein complements the activity of antibodies.

Complement can be activated early in infection, even before the development of specific antibodies. Some complement molecules known as zymogens are protease enzymes located within the gut that become activated by proteolytic cleavage.

Deficiencies of complement contribute to the development of certain diseases. Increases in complement indicate infection. Because complement in the brain contributes to synaptic pruning, a deficiency of one or more complement proteins can lead to inadequate pruning, whereas when complement proteins are increased, excessive synaptic pruning can occur.

## Complement Changes in Alzheimer's Disease

Although levels of complement are normally low in the brain, in vitro studies show that microglial, astroglial and neuronal cells can secrete most or all of the complement proteins when stimulated. Several studies show a three-fold increase in complement proteins C1q, C3, and C4 in the brains of subjects with AD compared to normal controls (Morgan 2017). In the brains of patients with AD, complement has found aggregated around amyloid plaque deposits.

In addition, the complement protein clusterin/apolipoprotein J has been found to be elevated in the blood of subjects with mild cognitive impairment. Clusterin is associated with atrophy of the entorhinal cortex and rapid clinical progression in AD. The subjects in the studies who went on to develop overt Alzheimer's disease exhibited an increase in clusterin levels as their disease progressed. Elevated levels were likewise predictive of greater fibrillar amyloid beta in the medial temporal lobe (Thambisetty et al. 2010).

## Acute-Phase Reactants

At the first signs of acute or chronic injury, infection, trauma, systemic autoimmune disease, or infarction, various proteins assemble to help launch an effective immune response. These proteins, which are called acute-phase reactants, are mobilized by acute-phase reactant cytokines. Acute-phase reactants also include platelets, complement, fibrinogen, C-reactive proteins, haptoglobin, ferritin, and other proteins. Normally present in the blood at levels that maintain health or a state of homeostasis, acute-phase reactants can either increase or decrease in concentration by at least 25 percent of their baseline levels.

## Cytokines

Cytokines are water-soluble, biologically active effector molecules that are primarily produced by CD4+ T lymphocytes as well as enteric neurons and glia (Yoo and Mazmanian 2017). As acute-phase reactants in infection or injury, cytokines play a role in cell signaling and modulating immune activities. Capable of being produced in nearly all nucleated cells if the need arises, cytokines act on both neighboring cells (paracrine effect) and cells that sent the signal (autocrine effect).

Cytokines function to direct cell trafficking, or movement of immune cells, to a specific area of the body, and they modulate the response appropriately. For instance, some cytokines promote inflammation (pro-inflammatory cytokines), whereas other cytokines reduce inflammation (anti-inflammatory cytokines). A careful balance between these two subtypes ensures that there will be a rapid destruction of the offending pathogens and that the inflammatory process will quickly end. In AD, imbalances in cytokine levels lead to a persistent neuroinflammatory process that results in conditions of neurodegeneration.

Chemokines are a specific type of cytokine released by infected cells. Infected host cells release chemokines into the circulation in an effort to initiate and strengthen the immune response and to alert neighboring cells to the infectious threat.

The interleukin (IL) cytokine subtype, one of the most prominent cytokines, gets its name from the fact that interleukins are secreted by and act on leukocytes. Other important types of cytokines, such as tumor necrosis factors (TNFs), are known to increase cell apoptosis (programmed cell death). The interferons (IFNs) can activate natural killer cells and macrophages, whereas transforming growth factors (TGFs) can result in phenotypic transformation and act as negative autocrine (affecting neighboring cells) growth factors.

Alzheimer's disease researchers from Greece have observed that increased levels of the pro-inflammatory cytokines may suspend the normal phagocytosis (engulfment and destruction) of amyloid beta in the brains of patients with AD. This result, in turn, interferes with the effective removal of plaque from microglia and promotes an inflammatory astroglial cell assault and neural death (Stamouli and Politis 2016).

A number of cytokine-related genes have been discovered. Polymorphisms that affect these genes and are seen in AD are described in Chapter Eleven.

## Cytokines in Alzheimer's Disease

In 2009, Kaori Morimoto and her colleagues at the Sun Health Research Institute in Japan measured cytokine levels in different regions of the brain in normal control subjects, in patients without dementia but with cellular signs of AD, and in patients with overt AD. These researchers found significant differences in IL-1 beta, 10, 13, 18, and 33, TNF alpha converting enzyme (TACE), and TGF beta2 mRNA expression between normal patients without dementia but signs of pathology and patients with overt AD. Their results show that these particular cytokines are more mobilized in the later AD stages, when a significant cognitive decline develops, than in the early stages, when housekeeping cytokines (going about their routine duties) are keeping things under control (Morimoto et al. 2013).

Agnes Pirker-Kees and her team at the Medical University in Vienna found that inflammation in AD was not limited to the central nervous system. The researchers tested peripheral blood samples from patients with AD and normal controls and found evidence of a strong pro-inflammatory response in patients with AD. These changes included activated glial cells, activated T cells, and increased levels of IL-6, IL-1, TNF-a, IFN-gamma, and IL-17 AD consisting of an increase of activated CD4+ lymphocytes with surface expression of the immune system markers HLA-DR and CCR5, along with an increased number of circulating lymphocytes producing IL-17, IL-6, and IFN-gamma, while total amounts of CD4+ and CD8+ cells were not altered in AD (Pirker-Kees et al. 2013).

With advances in mRNA sequencing, more recent studies have demonstrated a number of other significant cytokine changes in AD that point to a prolonged pro-inflammatory effect. For instance, to date twenty-three single-nucleotide polymorphisms involving thirteen cytokines have been found (Zheng et al. 2016). Many cytokines, including IL-1 beta, IL-6, and TGF-beta, have been found localized around the amyloid plaque deposits in the brains of AD patients. Researchers have studied cytokine concentrations in the brain and spinal fluid of AD patients. These studies indicate that several pro-inflammatory cytokines (particularly IL-1 beta, IL-6, and TNF-alpha), as well as the anti-inflammatory receptor antagonists IL-1 receptor antagonist and IL-10, which block the receptors that would normally be activated by anti-inflammatory cytokines, are elevated in AD, causing persistent inflammation (Zheng et al. 2016).

## Immunosenescence

Dramatic aging-related changes to the immune system begin in the sixth decade of life, and over time these changes progress to immunosenescence, a condition in which the immune system can no longer launch an effective immune response and prevent infection. Immunosenescence affects both innate and adaptive immunity. Most notably, the function and expression of cell receptors for immune contributions wanes, which causes a decreased response to pathogens and weakened adaptive immunity. Simultaneously, in aging the switch is to a pro-inflammatory response to damaged and dying cells, a process referred to as inflammaging. As the innate immune system takes over, pro-inflammatory cytokines such as TNF-alpha rise.

As people age, their weakened immune systems cause greater susceptibility to bacterial infection. Even healthy older individuals are more vulnerable to more severe bacterial and viral infections. Sepsis caused by severe infection can cause permanent cognitive dysfunction among this age group in particular. Scores from the mini-mental state examination are typically below 24, indicating a common finding of dementia in elderly patients with sepsis (McManus and Heneka 2017). Studies also show that the incidence of infection (particularly pneumonia, lower respiratory tract, and urinary tract infections) is higher in AD patients than in normal age-matched control subjects (Natawala et al. 2008).

Studies show an altered immune profile in the aged brain characterized by an increase in the production and release of pro-inflammatory immune cells and their associated chemicals, an increase in reactive oxygen species, and an increase in protein aggregation processes, which are all associated with neurodegeneration.

Most changes can be attributed to alterations in the activation status of microglia, which is referred to as microglial dystrophy (Kabba et al. 2018). The morphological features of these impaired microglia include loss of cytoplasmic processes, presence of cytoplasmic beading, and instances of cytoplasmic fragmentation. These alterations ultimately lead to a decreased response to pathogens and the development of several age-related diseases, including Alzheimer's disease, diabetes and cardiovascular disease (Sellami et al. 2018).

Aging also leads to involution and atrophy of the thymus gland, with a decline in naïve T and B lymphocytes, an accumulation of memory cells, and decreased antibody production. Inflammation is enhanced by the release of more pro-inflammatory cytokines. In aging, macrophages increase their pro-inflammatory activities, releasing increased amounts of TNF-alpha and IL-12, which can accelerate tissue damage (Sellami et al. 2018). Aging may also result in the proliferation of oral anaerobic bacteria, which can affect the gut microbiome. Evidence indicates that the microbiome influences health and how well people age (Shoemark and Allen 2015).

The immune system's eventual deterioration depends on a number of factors, including genetics and environmental influences such as diet, nutrition, exposure to infectious agents and chronic physical stress. A common genetic influence is the presence of HLA-DR4, a major histocompatibility complex (MC) Class II haplotype seen in individuals with rheumatoid arthritis (RA), polymyalgia rheumatica, type 1 diabetes, and other autoimmune conditions. Instead of having the phenotype CD4+ CD28+, which has been found in the synovial fluid of individuals with RA, these individuals lose the co-stimulatory CD28+ molecule. This loss is recognized as a reliable marker of aging in T cells. Individuals with this haplotype have shortened telomere sequences, which affects naïve unprimed T cells and an increase in inflammatory immunosenescent T cells. Researchers propose that aged T cells may be a critical effector cell in the process of RA development rather than a consequence of RA (Weyand and Goronzy 2016).

Old T cells lose their ability to repair cells with damaged DNA, have reduced signaling functions, and generate increased amounts of reactive oxygen species due to their impaired metabolisms. The loss of robust competent T cells contributes to the chronic inflammatory process.

Several longevity and genetic researchers have found that certain foods and dietary supplements can lead to genetic changes that help preserve immune function (see Chapter Twelve). Researchers have also found that exercise and training can delay immunosenescence and improve immune function. Elderly individuals are able to recruit T lymphocytes and NK cells in response to an acute bout of exercise. While physical exercise training programs do not result in complete restoration of the senescent immune system, improvement is seen with continual training, particularly in response to the function and number of circulating NK cells. Studies show that highly conditioned elderly individuals seem to have a relatively better-preserved immune system (Sellami et al. 2018). See Chapter Twelve for more information.

Researchers have also found that in immunosenescence the neuroprotective role of immune cells may be impaired due to the increased expression of the IL-6 receptor, which has previously been associated with cognitive deficits (Kabba et al. 2018). In addition, a decline in cognition may be related to the increased vulnerability of the hippocampus with age, as the hippocampus is involved with learning, memory, and planning.

The stepwise interactions of microglia, neurons, and astrocytes are adversely affected by inflammaging, which is thought to also contribute to neuroinflammation. Increased inflammatory markers by astrocytes and increased protein aggregate formation by oligodendrocytes likewise contributes to the transition from neuroinflammation to neurodegenerative disease. Neuroinflammation is demonstrated in the brains of AD patients through activated microglial cells, reactive astrocytes, and complement deposits in the vicinity of amyloid plaques.

In the early stages of AD, the immune system cells are able to efficiently clear amyloid beta via microglial housekeeping with the help CD14 and toll-like receptor (TLR)–promoting lymphocytes. The production of amyloid oligomers during APP processing, however, significantly increases amyloid production while destroying synapses. The combination of excessive microglial stimulation and neuroinflammatory signaling through pro-inflammatory cytokines and reactive oxygen and nitrogen species leads to the destruction of neurons and glial cells. Phagocytosis is impaired due to reduced signaling capabilities, resulting in accumulations of Aβ-42.

## Neurodegeneration

Neuroinflammation, attributed to immunosenescence or directly as a result of pathogens, is caused by a persistent microglial activation that recruits the activation of astrocytes. Excessive glial cell activation can result in disruptions in the BBB. This disruption leads to the entry of pathogens as well as other immune cells and their products, including toxic lipopolysaccharides from the gut microbiota and peripheral blood. Although they have different chemical structures, lipopolysaccharides and amyloids produced by bacteria can react with the same toll-like receptor (TLR2/TLR1) system as Aβ-42.

This situation allows these proteins to strongly activate the production of pro-inflammatory cytokines, particularly IL-17 and IL-22. A need to inhibit the development of neurodegeneration led to the first use of fecal microbiota transplants to treat infection with *Clostridium difficile*. Fecal microbiota transplants are also used in several autoimmune diseases, including multiple sclerosis. The hope in AD is to develop treatments that treat gut dysbiosis in a similar way, enabling the cycle leading to neurodegeneration to be halted (Sochocka et al. 2018).

Neurodegeneration is a disease process characterized by neuronal destruction and impaired production of new neurons and their extensions. Leslie Crews and Eliezer Masliah write that axonal pathology and the loss of synapses are probably key features in the development of dementia in neurodegenerative disorders (Crews and Masliah 2010). In Alzheimer's disease, the process of neurodegeneration is triggered by neuroinflammation that initially causes synaptic damage, which is followed by neuronal loss. Recent evidence suggests that alterations in the production of new neurons (neurogenesis) in the hippocampus also contribute to pathology, as the part of the BBB covering the hippocampus is the first area of the BBB to show signs of vulnerability. Studies also show that synaptic loss is likely the result of accumulations of amyloid oligomers rather than amyloid fibrils.

Amyloid oligomers have various mechanisms that allow them to cause synaptic damage: by forming pores with channel activity, altering glutamate receptors and causing excitotoxicity of neural circuits, inducing mitochondrial dysfunction, and causing lysosomal failure and thereby causing signaling failures. These mechanisms all tie in with the alterations in signaling proteins, including several different kinase enzymes that are involved in the progression of neurodegeneration that results in AD (Crews and Masliah 2010).

Neurogenesis in the healthy nervous system occurs throughout life in the olfactory bulb, the subventricular zone, and the dentate gyrus (DG) of the hippocampus. In the mature brain, neurogenesis in the DG is influenced by environmental and genetic factors and is associated with synaptic plasticity, memory and learning.

## Summary

Changes in the brain and peripheral blood of patients with Alzheimer's disease provide evidence of a persistent neuroinflammatory response that simultaneously prevents the normal removal of amyloid plaque deposits. Persistently activated glial cells accompanied by alterations in cytokines and complement lead to a cascade of events that result in neural destruction and neurodegenerative disease.

Normal immune alterations related to aging (immunosenescence) can account for some of the observed inflammatory changes. However, in Alzheimer's disease the increase in pro-inflammatory acute-phase reactant cytokines is more indicative of an underlying infectious disorder, with changes possibly accelerated by vascular defects and disruptions to the blood-brain barrier, which facilitates the entry of gut microbes and their products into the central nervous system.

# FIVE

# Stages and Pathology
# of the Disease

Besides the alterations in gut flora, the presence of microbes in the brain, and the changes seen in immune system cells and chemicals, other factors have been found to be involved in the pro-inflammatory pathology that leads to Alzheimer's disease (AD). Other physiological changes involved in the development of AD include poorly functioning mitochondria, defects in the blood-brain barrier, alterations in blood vessels, defects in apoptosis, defects in autophagy and lipopolysaccharide alterations.

Despite the many technological advances that enable researchers to study every facet of the AD brain, the question of whether AD is a pure disease or a combination of two or more conditions with cortical and subcortical cognitive changes remains under debate (Fülöp et al. 2018, "Infection Hypothesis"). Whether the neurodegeneration seen in the brains of patients with sporadic AD occurs as a result of immunosenescence or is a combination of vascular disease and infection in AD, the clinical picture remains the same. However, treatment options (including lifestyle interventions) can carry different weight depending on the causes.

This chapter describes the different stages of Alzheimer's disease and the battery of tests used in its diagnosis. It includes the role of dysfunctional mitochondria, defects in the blood-brain barrier, the contributions from vascular defects, the defects in apoptosis and autophagy that contribute to disease, and the lipopolysaccharide abnormalities seen in AD.

## Alzheimer's Disease Stages

While the advances gained from neuroimaging procedures, genetic studies and protein biomarkers paint a clearer picture of the stages in AD, two decades ago the stages were based primarily on cognitive function tests and activities of daily living (ADL). These parameters were sometimes difficult to gauge in individuals with hearing or sight impairments or who had other undiagnosed medical conditions affecting the results.

## Mini-Mental Status Examination (MMSE)

The MMSE is the most widely used evaluation tool for measuring the severity of dementia. Patients with mild dementia have a score of 22–30, with moderate dementia receiving a score of 11–21, and severe dementia 0–10. Patients with good cognitive abilities have scores higher than 30. The MMSE results are based on assessments of orientation, memory, attention and calculation, language, ability to write a sentence, ability to follow commands and to write a sentence, and ability to copy a drawing. Because the subject's education level can affect these scores, some researchers have proposed using a lower cutoff of 23 for individuals with at least eight years of education, and education is often taken into consideration when evaluating scores. A criticism of the MMSE is that results can vary based on the mode of test administration, which can influence the score.

## Reisberg's Seven Stages of Alzheimer's Disease

The seven stages of Alzheimer's disease (which are also known as the FAST—Functional Assessment Staging Scale) were first described in the early 1980s by Barry Reisberg, MD, clinical director of the New York University School of Medicine's Silberstein Aging and Dementia Center. This model was first introduced as a diagnostic tool in the early 1990s and is still in use. The stages are based on one's ability to perform the activities of daily living. These stages include the following:

Stage 1. No impairment (normal ADL); no memory problems or symptoms

Stage 2. Very mild cognitive decline; individual notices memory lapses, but family members and co-workers aren't aware of symptoms

Stage 3. Mild cognitive decline, with some individuals diagnosed with early-stage AD; inability to choose correct words; difficulty remembering names; losing or misplacing objects

Stage 4. Moderate cognitive decline (mild or early-stage AD); forgetfulness of recent events or communication; inability to perform challenging mental math problems; mood changes

Stage 5. Moderately severe cognitive decline (moderate or mid-stage AD); noticeable gaps in memory and thinking; help needed with ADL; inability to recall their address, phone numbers or educational background

Stage 6. Severe cognitive decline (moderately severe or mid-stage AD); worsening of memory; changes in personality; extensive help needed with ADL; inability to recall recent activities; able to remember own name but not background; can recognize familiar versus unfamiliar faces but not their significance

Stage 7. Very severe cognitive decline (severe or late-stage AD); inability to respond to environment or converse; may need help eating or using the toilet; muscles grow rigid

In Reisberg's Global Deterioration Scale (published in 1983), based on his previous work, stages 1–3 indicate pre–Alzheimer's disease and stages 4–7 are recognized as Alzheimer's disease. Other early classification systems characterize AD as having three stages: an early stage, a middle stage, and a late stage.

Newer classifications list the stages as preclinical or prodromal or subjective memory impairment when imaging tests or markers show signs suggestive of AD in the absence of overt cognitive symptoms; mild cognitive impairment (MCI) when symptoms of memory impairment first begin to appear; and overt AD when neuroinflammation results in neurodegenerative disease with memory impairment. Around 50–60 percent of individuals with MCI have prodromal AD, indicating that they have underlying AD pathology and will progress to AD with dementia (Blennow and Zetterberg 2015; Livingston et al. 2017).

## Prodromal and Preclinical Alzheimer's Disease

In 2007, prodromal AD (also referred to as MCI due to AD) was defined by the presence of episodic memory disturbances and one or more abnormal AD biomarkers. These biomarkers include presence of amyloid beta (Aβ) and tau proteins in spinal fluid; volumetric MRI showing brain atrophy; and positron emission tomography (PET) detection of brain amyloid (Blennow and Zetterberg 2015). However, tau protein is elevated in the spinal fluid of patients with stroke, Creutzfeldt-Jakob disease, and encephalitis.

Preclinical AD occurs when an individual exhibits Alzheimer's pathogenic changes but shows no evidence of memory impairment. These pathogenic changes include extracellular deposits of Aβ protein and intracellular accumulation of tau protein. The purpose of this classification is to identify individuals at a high risk of progressing to dementia, which gives them an opportunity to participate in treatment trials (Livingston et al. 2017).

The newer classifications are based on the premise that neuroinflammation occurs before the development of Aβ protein plaque deposits or neurofibrillary tau tangles appear.

## DSM-IV and NINDS-ADRDA Criteria

The *Diagnostic and Statistical Manual of Mental Disorders*, fourth edition (DSM-IV) criteria for a diagnosis of dementia require the loss of two or more of the following traits: memory, language, calculation, orientation and judgment. The National Institute of Neurological and Communicative Disorders and Stroke–Alzheimer's Disease and Related Disorders Association (NINDS-ADRDA) Work Group requires the presence of dementia that is first documented by clinical examination along with deficits in at least two cognitive domains, including absence of other cognitive disorders, absence of other systemic disorders, and progressive worsening of memory. If all criteria are met, the patient receives a probable diagnosis of Alzheimer's disease (Bekris et al. 2010).

## Protein Markers in Blood and Cerebrospinal Fluid (CSF)

The few tests traditionally used to help diagnose Alzheimer's disease are criticized because they lack specificity. Regional brain atrophy can be measured with structural MRI to assess neurodegeneration, and functional PET can detect hypometabolism as well as areas of plaque and tau. Cerebrospinal fluid (CSF) measures of amyloid beta (Aβ) peptide, total tau (t-tau), and hyperphosphorylated tau (p-tau) have greater specificity and are now established as diagnostic criteria for AD in prodromal and preclinical phases.

The CSF protein markers are more significant in the early stages of AD based on the premise that Aβ-42 builds up in the central nervous system before changes in tau occur. The presence of Aβ-42 alone in CSF indicates an earlier stage of AD. Tau and amyloid are seen in the CSF in moderate stages of AD and begin to clear as these proteins move from the CSF into the brain in the later stages of the disease.

Researchers at Mayo Clinic used four neuroimaging tests along with the CSF biomarkers to estimate the stages of AD. Using PET scans, Clifford Jack and his colleagues tested for 18-F-fluorodeoxyglucose (FDG)–PET to assess hypometabolism, tau PET, and amyloid PET to gauge brain accumulations of tau protein and Aβ, as well as structural MRI to measure brain atrophy in regions most likely to be affected in AD, along with tests for the APOE-ε4 allele (Jack et al. 2016).

Tests for hypometabolism and atrophy are not specific for AD, and the APOE-ε4 isoform is present in only a minority of patients with late-onset AD. Because tau is present in a number of other conditions called tauopathies (including Parkinson's disease) and amyloid protein is commonly seen in the brains of individuals without dementia, these categorizations, while helpful for confirming the diagnosis of study subjects, are unlikely to be used widely, especially given the many pitfalls involved in obtaining CSF samples for analysis.

## Artificial Intelligence Predictive PET Scanning

Artificial intelligence is highly effective at predicting AD development in subjects with mild cognitive impairment. Researchers at the University of California, San Francisco, trained a self-learning computer to recognize signs that are typically too subtle to see in 2,100 18F-FDG PET scans of the brains from 1,000 AD patients who participated in the Alzheimer's Disease Neuroimaging Initiative. Using this computerized technology, the researchers were able to accurately identify AD with 82 percent specificity and 100 percent sensitivity an average of 75.8 months before the time of their final AD diagnosis. By being able to identify AD patients early, therapeutic interventions can have a better success rate. Although this was a small study, it shows exceptional promise (Ding et al. 2018).

## Blood Tests for AD Protein Markers

No blood tests have yet been commercialized that can reliably diagnose AD, although the blood test for neurofilament light chain described in the next section may soon be available. Markers of acute-phase reactants can also be helpful for indicating an inflammatory process, but results may be unreliable in patients with deficiencies in immune function. After laboring ten years to find proteins to help diagnose AD, one team of researchers discovered that tests for complement factor H (CFH) and alpha-2-macroglobulin (α2M) were reasonably helpful, but with a sensitivity of only 62 percent and a specificity of 60 percent (Shi et al. 2018).

Other proteins these researchers investigated include clusterin, complement C3, gamma-fibrinogen, serum albumin, complement factor-I, alpha-1-microglobulin, and serum amyloid-P. These proteins were associated with hippocampal atrophy, which can have other causes besides AD. Another four proteins investigated were complement component C4a, complement C8, ApoA1, and TTR, which demonstrated blood levels that could discriminate fast-moving from slow-progressing AD groups (Shi et al. 2018). However, these studies haven't been replicated when other researchers tested similar proteins.

The problem remains that many of these proteins are also found to be abnormal in other conditions. For instance, albumin is frequently low in elderly patients, especially malnourished individuals. Alpha-2-macroglobulin is produced in the liver and is elevated in a number of chronic liver diseases, kidney diseases, and diabetes. Decreased levels of alpha-2-macroglobulin concentrations are also seen in pancreatitis, rheumatoid arthritis, and multiple myeloma.

Because Aβ oligomers have been found to be extremely toxic to neurons, tests are being developed to measure blood levels of these oligomers, including dimers, trimers, dodecamers, and larger molecular weight species. Because synaptic destruction occurs before neuronal destruction in AD, researchers are also attempting to develop procedures to measure the pre-synaptic elements of the synapse SNAP-25, which is being studied in CSF.

### Blood Test for NfL

In 2016, Mathias Jucker and his colleagues at the German Center for Neurodegenerative Diseases discovered that an elevated level of neurofilament light chain (NfL) could be a possible indicator of early-stage Alzheimer's disease. To explore this premise, the researchers examined NfL levels in 243 people with genetic mutations that predisposed them to AD and 162 people without the mutation. The researchers found that elevations of NfL were pronounced in individuals with the mutations, and these elevations showed up more than 16 years before symptoms emerged. An early diagnosis, the researchers report, would be immensely helpful because current therapies are started much too late (Terry 2019).

### Blood Tests for Amyloid Protein and Tau

Researchers at the Brigham and Women's Hospital in Boston are in the process of developing a test for tau protein in blood. Testing a patient's blood would be less invasive than testing CSF, which requires a lumbar puncture. In May 2019, the 2002 Nobel prizewinner for chemistry, Koichi Tanaka, announced that he and his colleagues had successfully developed a test to measure amyloid protein in blood. Tanaka explained that by measuring minute traces of amyloid beta from a teaspoonful of blood, physicians can gauge the progression of Alzheimer's disease and identify people likely to develop dementia in the coming decades (Matsuyama 2019). Researchers have also found that low levels of tau and amyloid beta proteins in vitreous fluid (from the eye) are associated with high blood levels of tau and amyloid beta protein.

## Origin of Mitochondria

Evolution studies show that bacteria lacking a nucleus evolved into eukaryotes. Two individual eukaryotic cells working together successfully produced the first insects and plants and humans. Every cell in every eukaryote, including humans, contains a tiny mitochondrion (pl. mitochondria) derived from ancient bacteria. Essential for health, mitochondrial organelles receive oxygen from respiration, which they convert into glucose. Mitochondria produce 90 percent of the energy needed for an individual's organs to produce life.

Eugenia Bone writes, "Mitochondria are fundamental to our ability to be more complex than bacteria, and yet they descend from a free-living bacterium that lived in the ocean 1.5 billion years ago" (Bone 2018, 55). Over time, the originating bacterium lost the genes necessary to survive on its own and shifted its function to its host cell, thereby becoming an organelle: the mitochondrion. Through the matrilineal line, females pass those bacterial cells and their genes from mother to daughter.

## The Endosymbiotic Theory

If the bacterial origin of mitochondria sounds new, it's because the endosymbiotic theory didn't enter the mainstream until 1981 with the publication of *Symbiosis in Cell Evolution* by the University of Massachusetts Amherst biologist Lynn Sagan Margulis, who had studied earlier theories of symbiosis (interaction between two different organisms living in close association with benefits to both).

After studying the close relationship between prokaryotes and eukaryotes and their organelles, Margulis adopted the term *endosymbiosis*. According to this widely accepted evolutionary theory, cells are engulfed, but not digested. Consequently, cells live together in a mutually beneficial relationship, or state of symbiosis. Margulis was not the first to describe this theory, but she was the first to get it established in high school textbooks.

The American biologist Ivan Wallin was the first to suggest the idea that the eukaryotic cell was composed of microorganisms. This idea was very significant in the formation of the endosymbiotic hypothesis. In 1927, Wallin also explained how bacteria could represent the primary cause of the origin of species. Thus, the creation of a species can happen through endosymbiosis. Margulis adapted this idea to propose that the tails on sperm are derived from spirochetes, a theory that hasn't been as well accepted. Still, in support of her endosymbiont hypothesis, she found parallel examples in plant cells where chloroplasts exist as a second plant body that converts sunlight into chemical energy.

Studies of the DNA in chloroplasts showed the DNA of cyanobacteria (found in oceans and fresh water). As for human mitochondria, early studies suggested that their DNA resembles that of a species that includes the bacteria that cause typhus. Recent DNA studies show a small but essential portion of the genome found in *Andalucia godoyi*, a member of the core jakobids in the bacterial phylum alpha-*Proteobacteria*. Nevertheless, only about 10–20 percent of the mitochondrial genome is consistent with that of ancient *Proteobacteria* (Gray 2015). Based on the genome present, the human mitochondrion is of absolute bacterial ancestry, but the exact mechanism and timeframe for this evolutionary undertaking remain unknown.

What is known is that the tiny mitochondrion is distinct from any other structures in the eukaryotic cell. Resembling a bacterium, it has its own membrane and its own DNA. However, rather than being encased in the cell nucleus like the host's DNA, mitochondrial DNA is formed in a ring of genes that resemble the circular plasmids seen in bacteria. Mitochondria also have their own ribosomes that resemble the ribosomes found in bacteria. In addition, to divide, like bacteria, mitochondria first replicate their genes and then split in two. Furthermore, if an injury caused the rupture of mitochondria, the immune system would react to the contents just as it does in a bacterial infection (Bone 2018, 56).

The number of mitochondria in human cells varies depending on the type of cell. Red blood cells do not have mitochondria, whereas liver cells can have as many as 2,000, and cells requiring the most energy (such as those in the heart, retina, and brain) can have as many as 10,000. The prefrontal cortex is the area of the brain found to be most densely populated with mitochondria (Amen 2017, 84).

As for the protobacterial origin of mitochondria, it's widely proposed that as *Cyanobacteria* grew and flourished, they produced a toxic form of oxygen. This development allowed for the formation of a unique bacterium with the ability to survive and create tremendous amounts of energy. The probable spirochete bacteria that engulfed this new species utilized this tremendous energy to form the first mitochondrion, an energy-packed organelle now found in all eukaryotic cells.

## The Many Functions of Mitochondria

Mitochondria are some of the key organelles in maintaining cellular homeostasis (all parts working together to maintain health), metabolism, aging, innate immunity, apoptosis (programmed cell death that characterizes each cell), and other signaling pathways. Mitochondria vary in size, shape, and motility, but their structure and movement are always consistent with those of bacteria. Mitochondria are composed of organelles that continuously elongate by a process of fusion. They divide through a process called fission and undergo a controlled apoptosis or turnover called mitophagy. Sensitive to changes in the cell, they rely on their dynamic abilities to divide, repair, and self-destruct as needed.

The dynamics of mitochondria play crucial roles in metabolism, the differentiation of cells into specific types, and the development of cancer and neurodegenerative diseases, including Alzheimer's disease, Huntington's disease and Parkinson's, as well as autoimmune diseases, diabetes, neurobehavioral and psychiatric diseases, schizophrenia, amyotrophic lateral sclerosis, cardiovascular diseases and Friedreich's ataxia (Nicolson 2014).

In its lifetime, a single mitochondrion undergoes fission and fusion several times. When cellular mechanisms detect a damaged mitochondrion, they eliminate it via mitophagy. Mitophagy is also employed during periods of starvation, fertilization and red blood cell differentiation (Khan et al. 2015). In fusion, the mitochondria quickly exchange and equilibrate new components, including matrix metabolites, membrane components and mitochondrial DNA copies.

Mitochondrial dynamics and mitophagy are the two main pathways needed for high-quality mitochondria and cellular homeostasis. Disturbances in these two pathways cause mitochondrial dysfunction and represent the most common reasons for neurodegenerative disorders and cancers. A reduction in the synthesis of high-energy molecules such as adenosine triphosphate (ATP) is a characteristic of aging and of all chronic diseases (Nicolson 2014). Viruses exploit these mitochondrial disturbances to their own benefit, manipulating the cellular machinery to produce an intracellular environment ideal for viral replication by altering cellular metabolism, signaling, and survival, making way for persistent viral infection (Khan et al. 2015).

## Mitochondrial Dysfunction in AD

Mitochondrial dysfunction results from several different circumstances: (1) a loss of maintenance of the signaling system (the electrical and chemical transmembrane potential of the mitochondria's inner membrane); (2) disruptions in the function of the electron transport chain; or (3) a reduction in the transport of critical metabolites and nutrients into mitochondria (Nicolson 2014). Exposure to the 1800 MHz radiofrequency used in cell phones has also been found to cause oxidative damage to mitochondrial DNA (Xu et al. 2009). These changes cause reduced efficiency of oxidative phosphorylation and reduced ATP production.

Mitochondria are able to produce ATP by converting the energy of metabolites to reduced nicotinamide adenine dinucleotide (NADH) and transferring NADH electrons to both the electron transport chain and oxygen molecules while moving protons from the mitochondrial matrix to the intermembrane space. The resulting transmembrane potential uses the enzyme ATP synthase in its final step of producing ATP. The entire process results in reactive oxygen species and reactive nitrogen species byproducts. Another consequence is a controlled leak of protons, which reduces ATP production and has the potential to damage mitochondrial membrane lipids. Natural antioxidants such as glutathione are used to help reduce the effects of mitochondrial dysfunction.

According to Garth Nicolson, research professor in the Department of Molecular Pathology at the Institute for Molecular Medicine in Huntington Beach, California, several antioxidant components essential to this system need routine replacement and can be improved by using a variety of nutritional supplements described in Chapter Twelve.

With the aid of an electron microscope, mitochondrial dysfunction has been observed for more than forty years in the brains of patients with AD. Altered mitochondrial infrastructures, deficiencies of mitochondrial enzymes and reduced numbers of mitochondria in damaged neurons represent early findings. While initial studies showed structural differences, later studies showed functional differences.

Aβ peptides are a known cause of mitochondrial dysfunction and early on were thought to trigger the process leading to AD. In animal studies using mice, the degree of mitochondrial dysfunction in different areas of the brain correlated with the extent of Aβ deposits. In addition, synaptic neuronal mitochondria were more impaired than nonsynaptic neuronal mitochondria in the AD mouse models (Dragicevic et al. 2010). However, not all of the animal researchers agreed that Aβ was responsible.

Researchers at the University of Kansas became interested in the structural and functional deficits in the mitochondria of patients with AD. Knowing that either Aβ or overexpression of its precursor protein caused deficits in mitochondrial function, they questioned whether Aβ triggered the cascade of steps leading to AD. Consequently, they designed a study to determine whether Aβ drove the process leading to mitochondrial dysfunction or if mitochondria initiated a series of steps that leads to AD, taking into consideration previous research findings such as reduced cytochrome oxidase activity in the AD brain along with altered calcium homeostasis.

They found that mitochondrial and bioenergetics alterations could contribute to AD development and that Aβ may influence these alterations and initiate a secondary cascade of events. Their data supported the possibility of both primary and secondary mitochondrial cascades in AD, the second cascade being triggered by Aβ. They concluded that therapies targeting the mitochondrial dysfunction seem a reasonable next step (Swerdlow 2018).

Susceptible neuronal populations in the brains of patients with AD show that damage to the nucleic acid building blocks of protein is primarily limited to the cytoplasm. To researchers in Japan, this finding suggested a problem with mitochondria and chronic oxidative stress. Oxidative stress is also known to damage the proteins that make up neurofibrillary tangles and Aβ deposits. That the affected neurons showed no visible signs of degeneration also suggested more subtle cellular abnormalities.

The Japanese researchers designed a study to determine whether mitochondrial abnormalities are associated with vulnerable neurons in AD. The results showed major abnormalities in mitochondrial dynamics restricted to vulnerable neurons. Increased levels of mitochondrial DNA and protein were found in the cytoplasm. There was also a significant decrease in the number of mitochondria found in vulnerable neurons. The fact that abnormalities occurred in neurons with no evidence of neurofibrillary tangles shows that mitochondrial abnormalities are the first cellular pathological change to occur in AD. The study findings also suggest an intimate relationship between mitochondria and oxidative damage in AD (Hirai et al. 2001).

Oxidative damage is known to occur during the process of aging. The oxidative damage that occurs in patients with AD appears to favor neurodegenerative events. An inefficient mitochondrial base excision repair machinery that prevents the normal repair of oxidative damage has also been found to contribute to the mitochondrial dysfunction seen in AD. The susceptibility of mitochondrial DNA to damage is much higher than that which occurs in damage to nuclear DNA. The accumulation of oxidized mitochondrial DNA bases that occurs during the aging process increases the risk for sporadic AD (Santos et al. 2013).

## Blood-Brain Barrier in AD

Blood vessels are composed of two distinct cell types. Endothelial cells form the inner lining of the blood vessel wall, and perivascular cells (pericytes), which are smooth muscle cells or mural cells, cover the outer surface of the vascular tube. The blood-brain barrier (BBB) is a protective outer layer surrounding the central nervous system, composed of epithelial cells from the vasculature (arteries, arterioles, veins, venules, capillaries) of the central nervous system that works in concert with pericytes and astrocytes to separate components in the blood circulation from neurons. The BBB protects the integrity of the brain's ionic environment, an environment conducive to the precise movement of signals transmitted across cell membranes and for synaptic transmissions and remodeling as well as the production of new blood vessel and neuron cells. The BBB also protects the plasma composition from circulating molecules such as neurotransmitters and xenobiotics that are capable of disturbing neural function.

To preserve its integrity, the BBB consists of more complex tight junctions than are seen in other vascular tissue, along with a variety of specific transport and enzyme systems that help facilitate molecular traffic across the endothelial cells. The functions of the BBB are coordinated by a number of physical, signaling, transport, and metabolic properties possessed by the endothelial cells of the blood vessels. These properties are closely regulated by interactions with different vascular, immune, and neural cells that work together to keep the BBB functionally intact.

The semi-permeable membrane allows astrocytes and other cells to quickly release cytokines and other factors that modulate endothelial permeability. Large, water-soluble, and low-lipid-soluble molecules cannot easily pass through the BBB, although lipid-soluble molecules such as oil-soluble vitamins and certain drugs can rapidly cross the semi-permeable membrane. Molecules with a high electrical charge can cross the membrane very slowly.

In certain areas, the BBB is naturally weak, which allows substances to cross into the brain freely. These areas of the BBB are called circumventricular organs. These include the pineal gland, which secretes the hormone melatonin and other neuroactive peptides; the posterior pituitary, which releases the neurohormones oxytocin and vasopressin into the blood; the area postrema, which causes vomiting when a toxic substance is introduced into the blood; the subfornical organ, which regulates body fluids; the vascular organ of the lamina terminalis, which detects peptides and other molecules; and the median eminence, which regulates the anterior pituitary gland through its release of hormones. With age, the area of the BBB covering the hippocampus also weakens and shows increased permeability.

Aβ is introduced across the BBB easily when permeability is increased, and it can also enter the central nervous system through the vagus nerve. The receptor for advanced glycation end products (RAGE) allows for Aβ's reaction with cerebral blood vessels. RAGE allows for the transport of Aβ into the brain. In mice studies, increased levels of RAGE are seen in AD. The transport of Aβ from the brain to the blood circulation is carried out by low-density lipoprotein receptor-related protein.

The BBB has transport systems that allow molecules to reach neurons or exit the brain. Five main transport systems exist: carrier-mediated transport, ion transport, active efflux transport, receptor-mediated transport and caveolae-mediated transport. Carrier-mediated transport is especially important since it allows for the transport of nutrients to neurons, including glucose, nucleosides such as guanosine, amines such as choline, and vitamins. GLUT1 glucose transporter is particularly critical in Alzheimer's disease.

GLUT1 protein expression in brain capillaries in reduced in AD, and the surface area of the BBB available for glucose transport is substantially reduced in AD. Consequently, the brain in AD suffers from a continuous shortage of energy metabolism, which has been consistently observed in PET studies. While individuals with age-related cognitive decline prior to developing AD also have reduced glucose, the areas affected are in the right precuneus, posterior cingulate, right angular gyrus, and bilateral middle temporal cortices. In AD patients, the deficits are more pronounced and involve the frontal cortices (Zlokovic 2008). Studies show that the reductions in glucose uptake across the BBB may precede the process of neurodegeneration and brain atrophy in individuals with mild cognitive impairment.

## Injury to the BBB

A number of factors can injure the BBB and allow entry of undesirable elements. The BBB can be injured in conditions of hypertension; stroke; multiple sclerosis; infancy (although the BBB is present at birth, it may be still developing); increased blood osmolality caused by a high concentration of substances in the blood; microwave exposure; radiation exposure; infection; trauma; low oxygen levels (ischemia); inflammation; and neurodegenerative disorders. Toxins impairing the BBB include hypertonic solutions, organic solvents, surface-active agents, enzymes, and heavy metals.

Defects in the BBB can lead to a changed ionic environment, altered signaling homeostasis, increased permeability, mild vascular bleeds, impaired glucose transport, perivascular deposits of blood-derived products, cellular infiltration, degeneration of epithelial and other cells, and the entry of immune cells and pathogenic molecules into the central nervous system, processes that lead to neuronal dysfunction and degeneration.

While leaky gut syndrome and gut dysbiosis result in an intestinal microbiome that's out of balance and frequently accompanied by fungi and parasitic worms, which elevate levels of cytokines and other inflammatory markers, defects in the BBB allow these microorganisms and their lipopolysaccharides and amyloid proteins, as well as inflammatory compounds, to easily find their way across the BBB, where they initiate neurodegenerative processes that result in dementia. In patients with AD, therapies aimed at restoring the gut microbiota will lower the inflammatory products and amyloid deposits that slip through the BBB (Sochocka et al. 2018). Other therapies include repairing leaky blood vessels to help in repairing the BBB.

## The Role of Aβ Protein

Studies consistently show that the production of Aβ varies in response to immune system challenge and its healthy resolution. Because of its antimicrobial properties, Aβ production is produced in response to infection, with levels falling as infection subsides. Persistent and latent viral infections do not allow for Aβ production to stop. Intracellular accumulations of Aβ are released when cells die and then produce extracellular plaque deposits. Therapies that reduce Aβ are associated with higher infection rates because of the reduced antimicrobial protection. In AD, Aβ also works to seal leaks in the BBB.

Aβ plaques in the AD brain contain a variety of proteins and peptides, including albumin, fibrinogen, thrombin, immunoglobulin G, collagen IV, hemoglobin and hemin, which are unexpected findings in the brain. Researchers have proposed that because plaques in AD are associated with capillary blood vessels, the deposits may act as scabs that seal breaches in the BBB (Brothers et al. 2018).

Researchers postulate that individuals with AD have a heavier plaque burden that becomes more porous than in individuals without dementia. Cortical siderosis (a condition of iron deposits in neurons) is seven times more common in AD due to the release of red blood cells that are linked with Aβ. Thus, the removal of Aβ has been found to cause more micro-hemorrhages in patients undergoing treatments to remove Aβ.

Aβ also has the potential to help repair leaks in the BBB after trauma. In addition, deposits of Aβ may remain after the resolution of infection. As has been widely reported, Aβ deposits are commonly seen in elderly patients with no signs of dementia. These deposits may result from the role of Aβ in repairing the BBB.

## The Circulatory System

The circulatory system is a network of organs and blood vessels that transport blood, nutrients, hormones, oxygen and other molecules to and from the body's cells. The main organs include the heart (the cardiovascular system), lungs (pulmonary system), and the liver (portal vessels). In addition, the circulatory system moves lymph fluid to rid the body of damaged cellular debris.

The cerebrovascular system refers to the blood vessels that transport blood to and from the brain. The carotid arteries (along the front left and right sides of the neck) and vertebral arteries (along the spinal column) pump oxygen-rich blood to the brain. These arteries contain numerous branches and tributaries called arterioles that travel to specific parts of the brain, face and scalp. The vertebral arteries arise from the subclavian arteries and pass through the transverse processes of the cervical vertebrae before entering the cranium through the foramen magnum. At the pons, the right and left vertebral arteries join together to form the basilar (vertebrobasilar) artery. At the base of the brain, the carotid and vertebrobasilar arteries form a circle of communicating arteries known as the circle of Willis. The jugular veins transport blood back from the brain to the heart.

Both arteries and veins have branches called arterioles and venules, respectively. Capillaries refer to any of the fine branching blood vessels that form a network between the arterioles and venules and transport blood to the body's tissues.

## Vascular Changes in AD

Prior to the emergence of cognitive changes, blood flow to the brain (cerebral blood flow) is reduced in AD. Patients with the APOE-ε4 allele are known to have disruptions in functional MRI (fMRI) connectivity (blood flow correlations) before amyloid plaque deposits appear. Blood vessels isolated from brain bank specimens from AD patients are known to release numerous cytokines, chemokines, and protease enzymes compared to blood vessels from control subjects (Zhan et al. 2018). In mouse studies, the AD brain shows both reduced blood flow and increased BBB permeability before cognitive changes emerge. For these reasons, both cardiovascular disease and cerebrovascular disease (including hypertension and atrial fibrillation) are considered risk factors for sporadic AD (Zhan et al. 2018).

Small blood vessel disease of the brain has been estimated to contribute to as much as 50 percent of all dementias worldwide, including those attributed to Alzheimer's disease (Sweeney et al. 2018). Some of the vascular changes seen in AD are suspected of being related to the breakdown of Aβ and tau proteins or to disruptions in the BBB. However, researchers have found that the vascular changes and alterations in the BBB seen in AD occur before Aβ and tau changes are observed (Nation et al. 2019).

Daniel Nation and his colleagues at the University of Southern California conducted a study in which they tested 161 patients and found a correlation between damaged capillary blood vessels in the region over the hippocampus and early cognitive dysfunction, regardless of differences in the Alzheimer's disease biomarkers Aß and tau. In this study, capillary damage was examined with dynamic contrast-enhanced MRI, and cerebrospinal fluid (CSF) levels of the putative marker for capillary damage, soluble platelet-derived growth factor receptor-ß, were tested (Nation et al. 2019).

## Defects in Apoptosis

Apoptosis is a process of programmed cell death that occurs in multicellular organisms. Cells, whether single cells or groups, die through either necrosis (caused by external forces such as trauma, poison, or reduced blood supply) or apoptosis. In apoptosis, cells begin a process of suicide at a pre-programmed time. In this way, old and dying cells are eliminated as they're replaced with new cells. Apoptosis occurs during embryonic development, organ development, cell turnover, pathological conditions, cellular damage, and aging. For instance, during neural development a tremendous number of neurons are produced, more than needed for synaptic connections, and then reduced by half through apoptosis to ensure that only the healthiest remain.

Apoptosis is a highly controlled process that's normally under genetic control and dependent on the action of caspase enzymes. Caspases have several subsets depending on their function: initiators, effectors, and inflammatory caspases. Stimuli that lead to early apoptosis include exposure to hormones, chemotherapy drugs and toxins, radiation, and bacterial infection.

In apoptosis, cells show shrinkage, membrane changes, nuclear condensation, and DNA cleavage. This situation results in a separation of cell fragments, and a loss of membrane lipids, with the contents retained in the cytoplasm body until engulfed by macrophages (Parthasarathy and Phillipp 2012).

## CNS Infection

In infections of the central nervous system (CNS), apoptosis can follow several immune-mediated pathways. Stimuli that activate the process initially cause changes to the mitochondrial cell membrane. Depending on the specific pathway, numerous molecules can activate different genes and lead to the production of various cytokines. Infections of the CNS include meningitis (inflammation of the meninges), encephalitis, (inflammation of the brain), myelitis (inflammation of the spinal cord) and brain abscesses. Infections of the CNS are primarily caused by bacteria, viruses, protozoa, spirochetes and fungi. Bacterial and other infectious factors, toxins, and lipids released by microorganisms in infection can generate reactive nitrogen and oxygen species and trigger apoptosis, especially in the hippocampal region (Parthasarathy and Phillipp 2012).

The loss of neurons to apoptosis in infection can quickly cause severe neurological defects, including cognitive deficits, hearing loss, motor neuron defects, sleeping disorders and seizures.

## *Lipopolysaccharides*

Lipopolysaccharides (LPS) are endotoxins primarily found in the outer membrane of gram-negative bacteria. LPS levels in the blood of patients with AD are three times higher than levels seen in normal controls, suggesting a role for LPS in the development of AD.

Large molecules, LPS consist of an O-chain composed of many simple sugars attached to a small chain of sugar molecules and a fatty substance called lipid A (two molecules of glucosamine linked to a cluster of fatty acids). As an endotoxin, the lipid molecules in LPS cause many symptoms, such as fever, that are typically associated with infection. These symptoms can persist after the infection is treated due to the released LPS molecules. Infections caused by gram-negative bacteria include urinary tract infections, pulmonary infections, oral infections and wound infections, although any of the body's tissues can be infected by gram-negative bacteria. Without proper treatment, gram-negative bacterial infections can lead to sepsis.

Recent studies show that gram-negative bacteria can form extracellular amyloid protein. Furthermore, 16S rRNA (a genetic indicator of bacteria) has been found to be present in all human brains, with more than 70 percent of cases showing gram-negative bacteria. In Alzheimer's patients, besides being present in excessive amounts in the blood, gram-negative bacteria are found in red blood cells. In addition, LPS was found to be deposited in amyloid plaques, vascular amyloid deposits, neurons and oligodendrocytes in the brains of AD patients (Zhan et al. 2018).

Researchers at University of California, Davis, hypothesized that LPS acts on leukocyte and microglial toll-like receptor (TLR)-4 and CD/TLR2 receptors to produce nuclear factor-kappa beta-mediated increases of cytokines that increase Aβ levels, damage the immune oligodendrocyte cells and injure myelin, all findings present in the AD brain. Because Aβ protein causes expression of TLR4 receptors, LPS can create a vicious cycle that leads to the persistent neurodegeneration and disease process in AD (Zhan et al. 2018).

From their studies, the researchers concluded that AD is caused by several factors such as inflammation, oxidative stress, and lack of oxygen. The source of the inflammation has been unknown, but the high blood levels of LPS along with the presence of microbes in the brains of AD patients suggests that microbes and their lipopolysaccharide endotoxins contribute to neuroinflammation. Their studies, using Western blot analysis, showed LPS in the nuclei of neurons in the brains of AD patients. Studies of the hippocampus showed increased LPS along with multiple strains of gram-negative bacteria (Zhan et al. 2018).

Gram-negative bacteria can enter the brain through leaky gut syndrome and defects in the blood-brain barrier. LPS is known to injure vascular tissue and increase the permeability of the blood-brain barrier, allowing pathogens to enter the brain. LPS also promotes hyperphosphorylation and leads to the production of tau protein. The researchers concluded that LPS could contribute to all of the key pathological features of AD, including amyloid plaques, myelin injury, and neurofibrillary tangles (Zhan et al. 2018).

# Defects in Autophagy

Autophagy (Greek for "self-eating") is a type of intracellular apoptosis in which the cellular proteins and organelles are degraded spontaneously by lysosomes (organelles in the eukaryotic cytoplasm containing digestive enzymes) and recycled to produce more energy. Dr. Steven Gundry describes this process as the cells' recycling program, in which the cell literally eats the pieces it wants to get rid of (Gundry 2019, 50).

A homeostatic mechanism, autophagy is especially important in neurons because the brain relies on healthy neurons for optimal neural function. Autophagy involves a complex set of steps that clear misfolded or damaged proteins and defective organelles and remnants of discarded membranes. In the gut, autophagy causes a reinforcement of the intestinal lining, resulting in a reduction of inflammation.

In 2016, the Japanese cell biologist Yoshinori Ohsumi received the Nobel Prize in Physiology or Medicine for identifying the genes involved in autophagy and the steps involved in this mechanism (Nobel Prize Awards).

Defects in autophagy are thought to contribute to the neurodegenerative process in AD and other disorders. Autophagy-lysosome defects are seen early in AD and considered a significant contributor to AD development since autophagy is the major pathway for neuron degradation.

Normal healthy cells have low levels of autophagy. Autophagy is increased in conditions of stress, including nutrient starvation, infection, oxidative stress, and tumor suppression (Uddin et al. 2018). In aging, autophagy is reduced, resulting in a population of older, damaged neurons. Such dysregulated autophagy leads to the accumulation of proteins inside the cell. Excessive autophagy causes excessive neuronal destruction.

Researchers describe the process of Alzheimer's disease as one of inflammation and autophagy (Uddin et al. 2018). Aβ influences the expression and activation of several genes that initiate autophagy, and it is known that autophagy and inflammation interact with neurons and influence the severity of the inflammation, presumably causing a persistent autophagy. Studies show the accumulation of the vesicles discarded after autophagy, which primarily occurs in the cortex and hippocampus (Uddin et al. 2018).

# Summary

Several factors that can be linked to infection are known to contribute to the development of AD. These factors include mitochondrial dysfunction, defects in the blood-brain barrier, neurovascular defects, defects in apoptosis, effects of lipopolysaccharides, and defects in autophagy. While the role of infection as a cause of Alzheimer's disease is becoming increasingly clear, the characteristic physiological changes that accompany infection, which contribute to neuroinflammation and degeneration, make this premise likely.

# Six

# Herpes Viruses

This chapter describes the herpes viruses that infect humans and the studies that indicate how specific herpes viruses play a role in the development of Alzheimer's disease. Although they are members of the same species, the various individual herpes viruses cause different symptoms during infection, different periods of latency, and variability in their episodes of viral reactivation.

## *Viruses*

Viruses are acellular microbes, meaning that they lack a distinct cell. Virus particles, called virions, contain either DNA or RNA (unlike living cells, which contain both) surrounded by a protein coat called a capsid. Capsids are composed of many small protein units called capsomeres. The shapes of capsids vary, including polyhedral (many sides), helical (coiled tubes), bullet shaped, spherical, or a combination of shapes.

DNA or RNA genetic material, along with the capsid coat, is referred to as the nucleocapsid. In addition to the capsid, some viruses (including herpes) are surrounded by an outer envelope composed of lipids and polysaccharides. This viral envelope, which is derived from the fragments of the host's outer or nuclear membranes, is acquired by certain animal viruses as they escape from the nucleus or cytoplasm of the host cell by budding. Thus, herpes is referred to as an enveloped virus. Bacterial viruses (bacteriophages) may also contain a tail, sheath, and tail fibers.

The first appearance of viruses is unknown, but they are thought to have emerged on the Earth at around the same time as bacteria. The "escaped gene theory" is the most widely accepted premise for the origin of viruses. According to this theory, viruses were acquired as the genetic material escaped from living cells. Thus the viral genes are no longer under cellular control. Because viruses lack cells, they are considered non-living entities.

As obligate parasites, viruses rely on host cell energy and molecular machinery to replicate. Viruses strategically manipulate their hosts' physiology and metabolism to create an environment conducive for them to replicate. Consequently, viruses cannot replicate spontaneously. Their replication is under the direction of the host cell targeted by the virus after the viral RNA or DNA has entered it. Viruses lack the genes and enzymes necessary for energy production. Instead, they rely on the host cell's ribosomes, enzymes and metabolites to produce the nucleic acids and proteins that they need to survive.

The first step in their multiplication is attachment (or adsorption) of the virus to a cell that has the appropriate protein or polysaccharide receptors on its surface. For this reason, animal viruses infect certain organs and certain species—for instance, humans or dogs. Viruses can also cross from one species to another, as demonstrated by the simian immunodeficiency virus (SIV), a retrovirus that has long been known to infect African primates. Viral strains from two distinct primate species—SIVsmm in the sooty mangabey and SIVcpz in chimpanzees—are thought to have crossed species and entered humans, resulting in the HIV-2 and HIV-1 viruses, respectively.

In the viral reproduction that occurs in humans, the type of genetic material in the virus and its number of strands determine the pathway used for the production of more viral proteins and viral nucleic acid. In the final production step, new virions are assembled. Newly assembled viruses then leave the host cell in a process called release (in which they destroy the host cell) or by budding (a process that leads to the production of an enveloped virus).

Viruses are classified based on the following properties: type of genetic material (RNA or DNA) and the number of strands (single or double); number of capsomeres; size of the capsid; presence or absence of an envelope; type of host that it infects; type of disease it produces; target cell; and immunologic or antigenic properties (Engelkirk and Duben-Engelkirk 2015, 48).

Bacteriophages (phages) are viruses that infect bacteria. Like all viruses, they must enter the host cell to replicate. Bacteriophages are classified according to their size and shape and the type of genetic material they have, as well as the number of RNA or DNA strands.

Viruses have long been suspected of contributing to Alzheimer's disease (AD). One prominent clue involves the 1918 worldwide flu pandemic. Survivors of this epidemic were shown to have a higher chance of developing Alzheimer's disease and Parkinson's disease (PD), which also could have been related to their overtaxed immune systems. Another clue is the fact that amyloid-beta protein in AD and alpha-synuclein protein in PD are antimicrobial proteins that arise in response to infection.

Another clue is the fact that all of the genes associated with AD can be traced to the immune system and are involved in clearing tissue debris (left from infection, cell death and related insults). Lastly, activated microglial cells and astrocytes, which are found in the brains of patients with AD, are intimately related to the immune system, indicating that neuroinflammation (presumably resulting from infection or stress) drives the disease process in AD. However, control subjects with numerous amyloid plaques and tau tangles with no signs of neuroinflammation are often found to have normal cognitive function, indicating that neuroinflammation rather than infection may be the driving force (Weintraub 2019). In addition, elevated levels of amyloid protein in serum (amyloidopathy) are seen in several chronic systemic diseases, especially chronic infections like tuberculosis and leprosy, which are caused by *Mycobacterium* (Mawanda and Wallace 2013).

## Latent Viral Infections

Herpes viruses that cause cold sores are a good example of latent viral infections. In latent infections with *Herpes simplex*, although the virus remains present in the body's nerve cells, the cold sores recur intermittently and their viral production (and reactivation) is triggered by fever, stress and sunlight. In latent viral infections, the virus is limited by the responses of the immune system (for instance, the actions of phagocytes, antiviral proteins and cytokines such as interferon that are produced by virus-infected cells). Shingles is caused by reactivation of the latent *Varicella zoster* (chickenpox virus), which, when reactivated, becomes *Herpes zoster*.

# Herpes Simplex *Virus (HSV)*

*Herpes simplex* is a member of the Family *Herpesviridae* and predominantly targets the epithelial cells of the oral and nasal mucosa. HSV has two subtypes:

- HSV type 1 (HSV-1) commonly causes cold sores and occasionally genital herpes; HSV-1 is usually acquired in childhood through direct contact with mucosal secretions or skin lesions.
- HSV type 2 (HSV-2) usually causes genital herpes and sometimes infects the mouth.

HSV-1 is an enveloped double-stranded DNA virus surrounded by an icosahedra-shaped nucleocapsid. The tegument, which is located between the capsid and the viral envelope, contains 26 proteins that are involved in the HSV lifecycle. HSV-1 has two distinct lifecycles. During its active or productive cycle, new virions are produced and cause host cell death. During this stage, the HSV genes express alpha proteins that regulate the viral genome, beta proteins that are involved in viral DNA synthesis, and gamma proteins that contribute to the viral structure. During the latent lifecycle, the viral genome persists within the host cell, but no new virions are formed (Harris and Harris 2018).

The infection caused by HSV is referred to as herpes, and it affects the area near where it entered the body. Oral herpes causes cold sores on or near the mouth. Genital herpes, which is a sexually transmitted disease, affects the genital area, including the genitals, buttocks, or anal area. Herpes infections can also affect the eyes, skin, and other body parts. Lesions in herpes can range from sores to itchy painful blisters while the disease is active. Outbreaks of herpes occur several times a year, although over time they occur less frequently. HSV-1 affects about 68 percent of the adult population worldwide, although only 20–40 percent of those affected develop clinically evident symptoms (Acuña-Hinrichsen et al. 2019). During infection, HSV-1 interacts with several proteins that it employs to facilitate entry into the host neuron and move easily from the cell membrane to the nucleus and back.

HSV-1 initially undergoes lytic replication in epithelial cells and then moves to the cell body of sensory neurons and sets up a lifelong latency in the trigeminal ganglia (sensory fibrous extension of the trigeminal nerve that occupies a cavity in the dura mater, covering the trigeminal impression near the apex of the temporal bone). Here the virus sets up a latent infection with periods of reactivation in which the lesions characteristic of herpes emerge. The trigeminal neurons also project to the trigeminal nuclei present in the brain stem, gaining easy entry into the brain in active infection (Piacentini et al. 2014).

HSV-1 is a neurotrophic virus, which means that it has a propensity to infect neurons, and it moves easily from the oronasal cavity to the central nervous system. HSV-1 is known to establish latency in neurons when its gene expression is repressed. When gene expression is activated in response to cellular stress, the virus is reactivated, causing increased risk for AD. Once the viral genome enters the neuronal nucleus, two different processes can occur: productive viral replication or repression of the genes causing latency (Acuña-Hinrichsen et al. 2019).

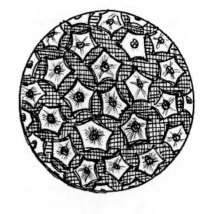

*Herpes Simplex* Virus (HSV).

In 2017, Ruth Itzhaki presented strong evidence indicating that HSV-1 plays a major role in Alzheimer's disease in individuals with the type 4 allele of the apolipoprotein E gene (APOE-ε4). According to Itzhaki, latent HSV-1 is regularly reactivated by various events, including immunosuppression, peripheral infection and inflammation. The consequent damage, which continues to accumulate, causes neuronal damage that leads to the eventual development of AD (Itzhaki 2018). Latent HSV-1 has been found in the areas of the brain affected by AD in a high proportion (70–100 percent) of brains from individuals with AD (Harris and Harris 2018). In addition, researchers have found that patients with HSV-1 who are treated aggressively with antiviral medications have a ten-fold reduction in their risk for senile dementia (Itzhaki and Lathe 2018).

Using population data from Taiwan (in which 99.9 percent of the population has been enrolled), Itzhaki found that the risk of senile dementia is greatly increased in patients who are HSV or *Varicella zoster* positive, with severe infections compared to HSV-negative subjects. Itzhaki began researching herpes viruses in AD in 1991. Since then, she and other researchers have noted that:

- HSV-1 DNA is found in the brains of both elderly control subjects and AD patients
- HSV-1 present in the brain of APOE-ε4 carriers confers a high risk of AD, and APOE-ε4 causes an increased risk for cold sores (clinical evidence of HSV infection); the APOE genotype modulates the extent of viral damage
- Intrathecal HSV-1 antibodies are found in aged subjects, showing that productive HSV-1 infection in the brain has occurred
- Amyloid beta (Aβ) and P-tau accumulation are found in HSV-1 infected cell cultures
- HSV-1 DNA is found in amyloid plaques of AD brains
- HSV-1 activates BACE1 via activation of PKR followed by phosphorylation of eIF2-alpha
- The antiviral acyclovir and related drugs, fucan, helicase primase inhibitor, and intravenous immunoglobulins (IVIG) greatly reduce the levels of Aβ and P-tau in HSV-1-infected cell cultures
- There is association of cognitive impairment in HSV-1-positive individuals
- HSV-1 viral load is higher in transgenic mice with APOE-ε4 genotypes
- HSV-1 affects amyloid precursor protein (APP) processing, causing increased production of amyloid beta (Harris and Harris 2018)
- HSV-infected neurons upregulate enzymes involved in the

hyperphosphorylation of tau, which leads to neurofibrillary tangles
* Amyloid beta fibrilization occurs when Aβ oligomer enfolds HSV-1 and binds its surface glycoproteins, which accelerates Aβ production and leads to a protective viral entrapment (Eimer et al. 2018; Itzhaki 2018)

Itzhaki notes that the viral concept does not preclude the theory that accumulations of amyloid beta and tau protein may be causes of AD. However, the viral concept suggests that these proteins accumulate because of HSV-1 infection. During antiviral treatment, levels of tau and Aβ fall. In particular, there is a larger decline in P-tau. Acyclovir inhibits viral DNA replication, and P-tau depends on viral replication, whereas Aβ does not require DNA replication. The decrease in Aβ is more likely due to the inhibition of viral spread.

Itzhaki explains that the increase in lysosomal load and impaired lysosomal function (which contribute to neurodegeneration) seen in early AD can be attributed to HSV-1. Infection and oxidative stress cause metabolic changes that result in an increased lysosomal load and abnormalities in autophagy that decrease the functionality of lysosomes. In addition, HSV-1 has been found in the DNA of enteric gut neurons, indicating that the virus is more widespread in the body than generally assumed. As part of the gut microbiota, HSV-1 has easy access to the brain in leaky gut syndrome and when defects in the blood-brain barrier occur.

Upon recognizing the virus via its pattern-recognition toll-like receptors (TLRs) on microglial cells, the innate immune system stimulates the secretion of cytokines such as interleukin-1 beta, interleukin-6, and tumor necrosis factor–alpha to produce an inflammatory response (Harris and Harris 2018). TLRs can either promote HSV-1 infection or hinder it depending on the levels of the various TLR subtypes. Deficiencies or absence of TLR2 reduce disease pathology, whereas an absence of TLR3 can quickly lead to encephalitis (Brun et al. 2018).

## Association with the Arc Gene

The activity-regulated cytoskeletal (Arc) gene encodes a protein that is critical for memory consolidation, neuronal morphology, and synaptic plasticity (change in the strength of synaptic connections induced by experience). A tightly controlled protein, Arc induces mRNA in response to neuronal activity. In HSV-1 infection, Arc mRNA is quickly transported to distal dendrites, where it may be locally translated before being degraded.

Researchers in Chile have studied the role of HSV in Arc induction and found that HSV infection significantly increases Arc protein levels. The researchers also found that by silencing Arc, infected individuals experienced a decrease in HSV-1 proteins and viral progeny, suggesting that Arc is involved in the lifecycle of HSV-1 (Acuña-Hinrichsen et al. 2019). Arc's particular importance is that it acts as a hub protein, meaning that it interacts with components required for AMPA receptor (AMPAR) recycling and with proteins involved with postsynaptic density.

The Chilean researchers are closely studying the relationship between HSV-1 neuronal infection and neurodegeneration. They have found that HSV-1 causes significant modifications of the neuronal microtubular structure, damage to the axonal and dendritic processes, and significant modifications in tau protein typically seen in neurodegenerative diseases. With mice studies, the researchers have found that there is an early increase in mRNA Arc in HSV-1 infection due to viral replication. This early increase in mRNA Arc also occurs during viral reactivation. However, ARC protein is stabilized during periods of latency (Acuña-Hinrichsen et al. 2019).

The role of HSV-1 in AD was first proposed in 1982, when researchers noted that damage to the brain tissue of individuals in the early stages of AD is identical to the same areas of the brain affected by infection with HSV-1. Although periodic reactivation of latent HSV-1 may cause no symptoms, symptoms appear when the immune system is weakened due to antibiotic use, aging, stress or immunosuppression. In these circumstances, the virus is freely propagated and migrates to several nerve cells, initiating a cascade of events leading to cell death and destruction (Sochocka et al. 2017).

## Fibromyalgia, HSV-1 and AD

Itzhaki describes several studies showing a link between fibromyalgia, HSV-1 infection, and AD. In one study, researchers treated patients with an antiviral drug in combination with a COX inhibitor, celecoxib. Celecoxib was used for its anti-inflammatory as well as its anti-herpes effects. Several herpes viruses, including HSV-1, are known to upregulate COX-2, which is needed for viral replication. Compared to patients given the placebo, those treated with the drug combination showed a significant decrease in fibromyalgia-associated pain (Itzhaki 2018).

Inflammation-related diseases or other pain-related disorders, such as headaches, are associated with an increased risk for dementia. A study of 41,612 patients ages 50 and older diagnosed with fibromyalgia were evaluated for their risk of developing dementia. Compared to controls, the patients with fibromyalgia had a 2.77-fold risk of dementia in the ten-year follow-up (Tzeng et al. 2017).

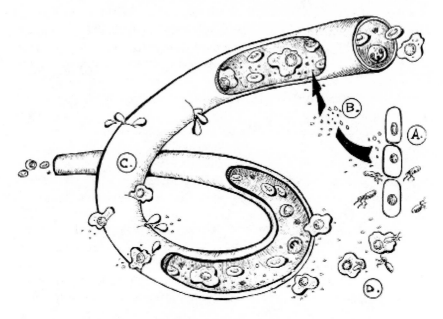

**Inflammation Response.**

## Epilepsy, Encephalitis, Viruses and AD

Seizure-like brain activity is associated with some of the cognitive decline seen in AD, and seizures are more common in AD than in the general population. Patients with AD have a higher risk of epilepsy, and 50 percent of AD patients are reported to have abnormal brain activity. Using intracranial foramen ovale electrodes, researchers detected clinically significant hippocampal seizures and epileptiform spikes during the sleep of patients with AD (Tzeng et al. 2017).

Paul Blocq and Georges Marinesco first described amyloid plaques in the brains of individuals with seizures in 1892. In fact, amyloid deposits are commonly seen in individuals with seizure disorders, and the plaque load is greater in seizure patients with the APOE-ε4 genotype. Both AD and epilepsy are associated with impaired cognition and an overlapping pattern of cellular neurodegeneration and hypometabolism in the temporal lobe (Lam et al. 2017).

*Herpes simplex* encephalitis (HSE) is a rare, often fatal, neurological disorder caused by HSV infection of the brain. While HSV is common in the peripheral nervous system, it rarely infects the brain. It's thought that latent HSV-1 in the trigeminal nerves becomes reactivated and ascends into the nerve fiber connections in the brain's limbic area. When HSV-1 enters the central nervous system, it causes brain inflammation. Acute HSE causes limbic pathology involving the hippocampus, temporal lobes, and frontal lobes, which are the same areas of the brain affected in AD (Harris and Harris 2018). Recent studies show that individuals with a mutation in toll-like receptor 3 (TLR3), which causes low or absent TLR3, are highly susceptible to HSV-1 encephalitis (Ewaleifoh et al. 2017). TLR3 has been found to offer protection against HSV-1-infecting neurons.

Symptoms associated with HSE usually develop gradually over several days, often with little warning. At the onset, symptoms include headaches, fevers, and seizures. Later symptoms include stupor and confusion or disorientation. After the initial symptoms begin to resolve, individuals with HSE may develop difficulties with speech and writing, lose their sense of smell, and experience memory loss. Some patients may also develop symptoms similar to those of meningitis, such as a stiff neck, convulsions and paralysis. HSE frequently causes epilepsy, and surgery for epilepsy causes a recurrence of HSE. In the last few decades, the use of antiviral drug treatment for HSE has reduced morbidity.

Francis Mawanda and Robert Wallace note that the high prevalence of HSV-1 in individuals 65 years and older makes the presence of HSV-1 in the brains of both patients and controls expected. In addition, the genes that influence the immune system's response to AD are the same genes that influence the immune system's response to HSV-1 infection. Still, the high levels of IgM antibodies to HSV-1 in AD patients, as well as the fact that HSV-1 DNA is found in 81 percent of AD samples compared to 47 percent in control subjects, make it likely that HSV-1 contributes to the development of AD (Mawanda and Wallace 2013).

### Herpes Simplex Virus Type 2 (HSV-2)

Studies to date have primarily focused on HSV-1 infection. However, HSV-2, as a known cause of severe oral lesions, may also cause the changes that lead to neurodegeneration and AD.

# Herpes Zoster *(Shingles)*

The *Varicella zoster* virus (VZV) that causes chickenpox is a human alpha herpes virus. When reactivated after a period of latent residence in the dorsal root ganglia (cluster of neurons in a dorsal root of a spinal nerve), VZV emerges as the *Herpes zoster* virus (HZV), which causes shingles. Chickenpox is a childhood illness that causes fever and pox-like lesions. Chickenpox was common until 1995, when the varicella vaccine became available for use in children. VZV is found worldwide but is more common in temperate regions.

Many older adults were exposed to chickenpox as children and are at risk for shingles when the VZV is reactivated, and this risk increases with age, stress, and immunosuppression, including corticosteroid therapy. Shingles can also occur after antibiotic use, as changes in the gut microbiome cause increased susceptibility to viral infection. Children as young as 19 months who have been vaccinated for chickenpox are known to occasionally develop shingles (Guffey et al. 2017). The shingles vaccine, Shingrix, is used to prevent shingles and minimize symptoms when shingles does occur.

VZV reactivation typically results in the development of *Herpes zoster* lesions, causing the painful skin rash that is a hallmark of shingles. The incidence and severity of shingles increases with age, immunodeficiency, organ transplantation or immunosuppressive drug therapy. HZV is a significant course of morbidity in solid organ transplant recipients, especially in patients who receive heart transplants, who may experience bacterial superinfection and chronic recurrences. VZV infections may also cause a debilitating post-herpetic neuralgia. Shingles is treated with the antiviral drugs acyclovir and valacyclovir as first-line therapies. Antiviral drugs interfere with virus-specific enzymes and virus production by either disrupting critical steps in viral reproduction or inhibiting the synthesis of viral DNA, RNA, or proteins. In particular, these drugs target the viral DNA polymerase enzyme responsible for viral replication. Resistance to these antiviral drugs is known to occur (Mercier-Darty et al. 2018).

A study from Taiwan matched 39,205 cases of subjects with shingles to control subjects without shingles, adjusting for age, sex, residence, depression and autoimmune disease, and ischemic stroke. In a follow-up period of 6.22 years, 4,204 patients had developed dementia. *Herpes zoster* was associated with a slightly increased risk of dementia. In addition, patients prescribed antiviral therapy for shingles had a reduced rate of developing dementia— about half the rate of the untreated group (Itzhaki et al. 2016; Chen et al. 2018). However, antiviral medications are also effective against certain bacteria (Broxmeyer and Perry 2018). The risk of developing AD has been found to be much higher in patients with *Herpes zoster ophthalmicus*, a condition in which the *Herpes zoster* virus infects the eye.

# Herpes Zoster Ophthalmicus *(HZO)*

*Varicella zoster* virus (VZV) is the only human virus that can replicate in cerebral arteries and produce vascular disease. This result primarily occurs in elderly and immunocompromised patients. VZV spreads transaxonally to cerebral arteries that feed the trigeminal nerve, particularly from the ophthalmic branch of the trigeminal nerve's afferent fibers. The trigeminal nerve is the fifth cranial nerve and is responsible for sensation and motor functions in the face.

The presence of VZV, which when activated becomes the *Herpes zoster* virus, results in even greater vascular inflammation and thrombosis, which have the ability to injure brain cells. VZV-related vascular disease has been previously found to potentially cause transient ischemic attacks, stroke, aneurysms, venous sinus thrombosis and arterial dissection. Compared to patients with *Herpes zoster* without eye involvement (HZV), patients diagnosed with HZO had a greater risk for stroke, a known risk factor for dementia (Tsai et al. 2017).

Researchers in Taiwan studied the records of 846 patients with *Herpes zoster opthalmicus* (HZO) using the Taiwan Longitudinal Health Insurance Database. These subjects were matched with 2,538 patients without HZO. Each patient was individually followed for a 5-year period to assess whether they received a diagnosis of dementia during this period. From this information, and using a using a Cox proportional hazards regression, hazard ratios (HRs) were calculated. The crude HR of dementia during the follow-up period was 2.83 for patients with HZO compared to patients without HZO. After the results were adjusted for patient characteristics and comorbid disorders, they indicated a 2.97-fold greater risk for dementia in all patients with HZO when compared to the control subjects. For males, the crude HR for dementia was higher, at 3.35.

At the end of the follow-up period, 4.61 percent of patients with HZO received a diagnosis of dementia compared to 1.65 percent of patients in the larger control group without HZO. The study's authors noted that psychological stress, aging, a poor social support environment, and adverse life events may contribute to both VZV reactivation and dementia. The study did not indicate whether patients used antiviral drugs (Tsai et al. 2017).

A number of studies show significantly higher amounts of various herpes viruses—particularly HSV-1, HSV-2, CMV, and human herpes viruses 6 and 7—in the brains of patients with Alzheimer's disease when compared to control subjects with no signs of dementia. Because these viruses are present in the majority of people, finding low concentrations of herpes viruses in the brains of individuals free of dementia is not uncommon.

## The Brain's Immune Response

The presence of chronically activated herpes viruses causes an accumulation of glial cells, the primary immune cells found in the central nervous system. In neuroinflammation, various immune system chemicals, pattern recognition receptors, along with cellular immune factors, increased amyloid beta, and pro-inflammatory cytokines cause a chain of events in which additional microglial cells and astrocytes are activated. This process prevents astrocytes from promoting neuronal survival. Consequently, activated astrocytes cause the death of both neurons and oligodendrocytes.

During acute infection, the brain's inflammatory reaction leads to repair of damaged brain areas. However, in chronic, persistent infection, neurons are destroyed. Normal mechanisms for repairing damaged neurons are impaired, and there is an increase in amyloid precursor protein (APP). The matrix metalloproteinases (MMPs), which play an important role in neuroinflammation, become activated in chronic infection due to the presence of amyloid beta protein molecules in blood vessels. Activated MMP molecules also contribute to neuronal death. The increased expression of MMPs in both brain tissue and blood of patients with AD is evidence of the inflammatory response that leads to neurodegeneration and the characteristic brain changes seen in AD.

## Human Herpes Virus

Viruses belonging to the *Herpesviridae* family that affect humans are known as human herpes viruses (HHVs). Named in order of their discovery, HSV-1 is also known as HHV-1, and HSV-2 is known as HHV-2. The *Varicella zoster* virus is also known as HHV-3, Epstein-Barr virus (EBV) is known as HHV-4, and cytomegalovirus (CMV) is HHV-5. While EBV and CMV and their association with AD are described in Chapter Seven, this section describes the associations of human herpes virus types 6 and 7 with AD.

In 1986, the human herpes virus type 6 (HHV-6) was the sixth herpes virus to be discovered as researchers attempted to discover new viruses with links to lymphoproliferative diseases. Since, the beta herpes virus HHV-6 has been found to have two distinct subtypes: HHV-6A and HHV-6B. Both subtypes are considered lymphotropic viruses with a high affinity for the CD4 T lymphocytes.

No specific diseases have been linked to HHV-6A, although reactivation of this virus in immunocompromised individuals is associated with a poorer prognosis. HHV-6B infection usually occurs in infants and children up to 24 months old and causes roseola infantum (sixth disease), a childhood disease causing a high fever for 3–5 days followed by a rash on the torso that spreads to the limbs as the fever subsides (Salvaggio 2018).

In patients with human immunodeficiency virus (HIV), HHV-6 may upregulate HIV replication, which speeds up the progression to AIDS. HHV-6 is also associated with reactivation of CMV and a more severe disease course. HHV-6 has likewise been implicated in the white matter demyelination that occurs in persons with AIDS dementia complex.

Human herpes virus type 7 (HHV-7) is transmitted mainly through saliva and infects nearly all children by the age of three years. Similar to HHV-6, it is known to cause some cases of roseola, although it is not clinically associated with any specific disease. It's believed that HHV-7 can contribute to other viral infections, and it's thought to be able to reactivate latent EBV infection.

Human herpes virus type 8 (HHV-8) is not associated with Alzheimer's disease, although it has a strong association with the connective tissue cancer Kaposi's sarcoma that can occur in individuals with HIV infection. HHV-8 is found in the saliva of many AIDS patients, although the infection rate is low in the United States.

Strong evidence suggests that both HHV-6A and HHV-7 may be associated with the development of AD. In a study conducted by the National Institutes of Health, researchers led by Joel Dudley at the Icahn School of Medicine in Mount Sinai, New York, found that many of the genes turned on in AD are identical to the genes that activate when the body is fighting a viral infection. The researchers then examined the RNA and DNA sequences of the brain of 622 patients with AD and 322 control subjects without dementia. They found that HHV-6A and HHV-7 were more common in the brains of subjects who died from AD. People reported to have more severe cases of AD showed the greatest signs of HHV. The study's authors emphasized that their results did not prove that HHV causes AD and that an infectious cause would not mean that AD was a communicable disease, but these results do suggest that the viruses worsen the disease course and exacerbate symptoms (Alzforum 2018; Daley 2018).

In a related unpublished mouse study, researchers exposed the brain cells of mice to these viruses. This led to a reaction or immune response that led to the formation of amyloid beta protein deposits. The researchers surmised that the activated viruses cause the buildup of amyloid plaque deposits that lead to the development of AD (Daley 2018).

## Summary

This chapter introduces readers to the microorganisms known as viruses, including their origin, replication, structure, and classification. In particular, this chapter focuses on the major herpes viruses and the infections they cause, including *Herpes simplex-1* and *Herpes simplex-2*; *Varicella zoster* virus and *Herpes zoster* virus, as well as *Herpes zoster opthalmicus*; and the human herpes virus types 6A, 6B, and 7.

Numerous studies have shown a close association between herpes viruses and the development of Alzheimer's diseases, and these studies are described in this chapter. In addition, viral particles and genetic material have been found in the brain tissue and plaques of patients with Alzheimer's disease in greater amounts than seen in elderly subjects without dementia. The immune response that leads to neurodegeneration in Alzheimer's disease is the same as the response seen in viral infection.

Herpes viruses have an affinity for targeting neurons. Although these viruses may take up a latent residence in the cells of the trimenal ganglia for years, upon reactivation they have easy access to neurons, setting the stage for Alzheimer's disease.

# SEVEN

# Other Associated Viruses and the Prion Connection

On average, during their lifetimes most people are infected with about ten different types of known viruses from a number of different families, including influenzas and rhinoviruses (which cause the common cold) along with one or more bacteriophages (viruses that infect bacteria). Both viruses and bacteriophages are common residents of the human gut, and prions are also sometimes present.

This chapter describes the common herpes virus known as cytomegalovirus along with several other viruses, bacteriophages and prions that have been found in the brain tissue of AD patients along with the role of these microbes in causing dementia. It should also be noted that studies suggest that a community of microorganisms, rather than one individual microbe, may be involved in triggering the development of Alzheimer's disease (Fülöp et al. 2018, "Infection Hypothesis").

## Cytomegalovirus

Cytomegalovirus (CMV) is a common virus that infects people of all ages. It is spread through direct contact with the body fluids of individuals seropositive for CMV (showing evidence of IgG CMV antibodies) with or without symptoms. Its most debilitating effects are seen in patients receiving transplants, unborn babies and congenitally infected newborns. Blood banks routinely screen blood obtained for transfusions for the presence of CMV to avoid giving CMV-positive blood to newborns and transplant patients. More than half of people older than age 40 have had CMV, which, like other herpes viruses, remains in the body throughout life and can become reactivated. CMV is more prevalent in areas where there is poverty and overcrowding, and blacks are more likely to be infected than whites.

In most cases, CMV infection causes mild symptoms of fever, swollen glands, fatigue, and sore throat. However, in immunocompromised and transplant patients, as well as infants, it has serious consequences, affecting the eyes, lungs, liver, esophagus, stomach, and intestines. Newborns infected with CMV often develop hearing loss and can have neurological, liver, spleen, lung, and developmental problems. CMV is also thought to potentiate symptoms in patients with coexisting viral infections. Individuals seropositive with CMV who are generally in good health frequently experience episodes of CMV reactivation (demonstrated by IgM CMV antibodies) with the development of overt symptoms, including symptoms affecting the central nervous system. These episodes of reactivation can lead to a higher percentage of CMV-specific T lymphocyte cells in older individuals.

CMV has found a unique way to replicate while skirting around the body's natural defense mechanisms. Researchers at the Gladstone Institutes–University of California, San Francisco, Center for Cell Circuitry discovered that CMV doesn't inject its own DNA into the host cell the way that other herpes viruses do. Instead, it links its viral DNA to proteins called PP71 and carries this compound directly into the cell. Once inside its host, CMV releases the PP71 proteins, which allows the viral DNA to replicate.

Realizing that the PP71 proteins quickly broke down, yet were needed for replication, the researchers conducted a study to determine how replication and infection continue. They discovered that while PP71 proteins are still present within the host, it activates E1 protein and recruits the protein to work in its place. This study could lead to therapies helpful for combatting CMV and other herpes infections (Langelier 2018).

## CMV in AD

In a study of blood, cerebrospinal fluid (CSF), and cryopreserved lymphocytes from 254 subjects in the Rush Alzheimer's Disease Religious Orders Study (ROS), CMV infection was associated with an increased risk of developing AD. Subjects included patients with no signs of dementia, patients with mild cognitive impairment, and patients with probable Alzheimer's disease.

Results showed that CMV IgG antibody levels, CSF interferon-gamma levels, and percentages of senescent T lymphocytes were highly associated with neurofibrillary tangles when compared to CMV-negative subjects. Subjects positive for CMV had high CSF interferon-gamma levels, and CMV-negative subjects did not show the presence of CSF interferon-gamma. In this study, HSV-1 antibody levels were not associated with CMV antibody levels and did not show the same immunological effects (Lurain et al. 2013).

In CMV-seropositive individuals, viral reactivation causes a decreased expression of co-stimulatory lymphocytes and an increased expression of CD57 molecules. These molecules are associated with an increase in senescent cells that are known to secrete the cytokines interferon-gamma and tumor necrosis factor–alpha, which are reported to cause deposits of amyloid beta proteins. In older individuals, CMV is associated with cardiovascular disease, and most previous studies have focused on CMV in vascular disease or vascular dementia. Since CMV is known to affect the central nervous system, CMV infection had long been proposed as a contributing factor in AD development. CMV is associated with the development of autoimmune diseases, conditions of endothelial dysfunction, and atherosclerosis (Barnes et al. 2015; Sochocka et al. 2017).

Another study published in the *Journal of Infectious Diseases* included 849 racially diverse subjects from the ROS study, along with subjects from the Rush Memory and Aging Project, which included older adults in the Chicago area, and the Minority Aging Research Study, which included older black individuals. The mean age of the subjects was 78.6 years, and their mean duration of education was 15.4 years. The researchers included a subset of 210 black patients from all three studies who had blood specimens available, an absence of dementia at the time of the blood specimen collection and at least two evaluations for cognitive decline (Barnes et al. 2015).

The researchers found that 73.4 percent of the subjects had IgG CMV antibodies, indicating past CMV infection. These included 89 percent of black subjects and 68.2 percent of whites. In addition, higher levels of CMV antibodies were seen in blacks at every age assessed. In an average follow-up period of five years, 93 of the subjects developed AD. The results showed that having CMV increased the risk of Alzheimer's disease two-fold and was associated with a faster rate of global decline (Barnes et al. 2015).

Another recent study indicates that the presence of CMV IgG antibodies did not influence the development of Alzheimer's disease. However, when CMV IgG occurred in individuals who also had antibodies to HSV-1, this interaction was associated with AD development, perhaps due to the increased immune system effects (Lövheim et al. 2018).

## Hepatitis C Virus

First discovered in 1988, the hepatitis C virus (HCV), a member of the genus *Hepacivirus* in the *Flaviviridae* family, is thought to have emerged in the United States shortly after World War II. An insidious virus, HCV usually causes no symptoms and infected individuals are often unaware of its presence until years later, when the damage caused by chronic infection is discovered. Only about 25–40 percent of patients develop jaundice in acute infection. Chronic HCV infection, which usually causes no symptoms, can lead to advanced liver disease, cirrhosis, and liver cancer, typically over a period of 14 to 28 years.

A single-stranded RNA virus, HCV mutates easily and has six major types with more than 51 subtypes characterized by alterations to the basic genome with variances in the nucleotide sequences as high as 30 percent. Because of the increased number of subtypes seen in Africa and Asia, HCV is suspected of originating in these parts of the world.

The hepatitis C virus is more widespread among individuals born between 1945 and 1965 because a rudimentary test to detect this virus in blood was not available until 1991, and more sensitive methods in use today were not developed until 1992. Consequently, blood banks didn't begin screening blood for transfusions until 1992. Prior to the implementation of the HCV blood test, individuals with elevated liver enzymes, jaundice and other symptoms of hepatitis who tested negative for hepatitis virus subtypes A and B were said to have non-A, non-B hepatitis. For this reason, and due to the fact that symptoms of hepatitis are often nonexistent and, when present, do not develop until weeks after infection, prior to 1992, blood used for transfusions and organs used in transplants transmitted HCV to many individuals.

HCV can be transmitted through childbirth, sexual intercourse, unsterilized medical instruments (including hemodialysis procedures), direct contact with fluids from infected individuals by housemates or medical personnel, intravenous or injection drug use, and, prior to 1992, transfusions of blood and blood products such as cryoprecipitate and organ transplants.

## Extrahepatic Symptoms

While HCV primarily affects the liver, because the liver interacts with so many other organs, it is considered a systemic disease. In HCV infection, symptoms in other organs of the body besides the liver (extrahepatic manifestations) often occur. HCV is associated with vascular disorders, autoimmune disorders, insulin resistance, type 2 diabetes, thrombocytopenia (condition of decreased platelets), head and neck cancers, cholangiocarcinoma (bile duct cancer), multiple myeloma, and lymphoma.

HCV is also associated with a number of neuropsychiatric disorders that are seen in up to 50 percent of cases (Adinolfi et al. 2015). The main HCV-associated neurological conditions include encephalopathy, encephalomyelitis, cognitive impairment, and cerebrovascular events, and the main psychiatric disorders include brain fog, fatigue, depression, and anxiety. Neuropsychiatric symptoms typically resolve with a sustained virologic response following interferon treatment. In addition, different viral sequences are seen in the livers and brains of affected individuals, suggesting independent viral evolution (Adinolfi et al. 2015).

## Hepatitis C and Alzheimer's Disease

While HCV primarily replicates in liver cells, the brain is also a suitable site for HCV replication, where the virus may directly exert neurotoxicity (Adinolfi et al. 2015). HCV within the brain can also trigger a cascade of neuroinflammatory and neurodegenerative changes, including alterations in signaling circuits and metabolic pathways that set the stage for AD development. In addition, both hepatitis B and C viruses have been found to manipulate and utilize changes in mitochondrial dynamics seen in these infections for the maintenance of persistent viral infection (Khan et al. 2015).

Perturbation in mitochondrial dynamics and mitophagy usually leads to an unhealthy pool of the mitochondria that result in an energy-deprived condition within the cell's cytoplasm that can eventually lead to apoptosis (cell death). Defective and damaged mitochondria generate reactive oxygen species, which can damage the remaining healthy mitochondria. Such defects impair the innate immune system's signaling, reducing its antiviral defenses. Chronic infection with both hepatitis B and C viruses has long been known to injure the mitochondria of liver cells, which leads to persistent infection, liver fibrosis, cirrhosis and hepatocellular carcinoma (Khan et al. 2015). Recent studies described in Chapter Five indicate that mitochondrial dysfunction is a key factor in the development of AD.

The association of HCV infection with dementia was first reported in the early 21st century. Since then, several published studies have investigated cognitive impairment in patients with HCV infection. Studies suggest that HCV may infect the brain, causing neurotoxicity, and chronic activation of the immune system could cause cerebral or systemic inflammation. HCV RNA and DNA have also been found in the nervous system tissue of individuals with dementia. HCV is likewise known to infect monocytes and macrophages and cross the blood-brain barrier. Even patients with mild hepatitis C have demonstrated activation of microglial cells and altered cerebral metabolism (Sochocka et al. 2017).

## *Epstein-Barr Virus (EBV)*

One of the most common human herpes viruses, Epstein-Barr virus (EBV), which is also known as human gamma herpes virus 4, causes infectious mononucleosis (mono) and several other illnesses. Although it is not always accompanied by symptoms, EBV causes a lifelong infection with occasional periods of reactivation.

EBV is spread through saliva and can be caused by kissing and/or sharing toothbrushes, silverware and drinks. Besides mono, EBV has been known to cause ear infections and diarrhea in children, Guillain-Barré syndrome, and certain cancers such as Burkitt's lymphoma and cancers of the breast, stomach, nose and throat. Mitochondrial dysfunction has been noted in EBV-infected cells due to elevated mitochondrial fission, which is thought to contribute to the metastatic behavior of EBV-associated gastric and breast carcinoma (Khan et al. 2015). Mitochondrial dysfunction is also associated with AD development.

EBV is diagnosed with tests for EBV antibodies to viral capsid antigen (VCA) IgG, VCA IgM, and Epstein-Barr nuclear antigen (EBNA). The presence of VCA IgG antibodies indicates that an EBV infection has occurred at some time recently or in the past. The presence of VCA IgM antibodies and the absence of antibodies to EBNA mean that the infection has occurred recently. Conversely, the presence of antibodies to EBNA means that the infection occurred in the past, as antibodies to EBNA develop six to eight weeks after the onset of infection and remain positive for life.

## EBV and Alzheimer's Disease

EBV has been isolated from the brains of patients who died of AD, and studies of patients who developed clinically evident AD show significantly elevated levels of EBV antigens. However, further studies are needed before EBV can be considered a definitive cause of AD.

One small Korean study from 2017 suggested that having a chronic infection with EBV can contribute to cognitive decline in elderly patients. The researchers evaluated plasma levels of IgG EBV in elderly patients with normal cognitive function to assess any differences in these levels in individuals who went on to develop mild cognitive impairment (MCI) compared to those who remained free of cognitive impairment in a two-year follow-up period. The individuals who developed MCI exhibited elevated levels of anti–EBV IgG antibodies in the follow-up compared to their initial levels, suggesting periods of reactivation and chronic infection, whereas the individuals who had preserved cognitive function had levels that had not significantly changed (Shim et al. 2017).

In addition, the two-year follow-up study discovered elevated anti–EBV IgG levels and found that they were significantly associated with Clinical Dementia Rating scales and total scores in the Consortium to Establish a Registry for Alzheimer's Disease battery of tests in the individuals who had progressed to MCI (Shim et al. 2017). These results suggest the need for more studies to evaluate the role of EBV infection in AD.

## The Human Immunodeficiency Virus (HIV)

The human immunodeficiency virus (HIV) is a lentoretrovirus belonging to the *Retroviridae* family, and it is the cause of Acquired Immune Deficiency Syndrome (AIDS). The associated HIV neurocognitive disorder (HAND) commonly occurs in HIV infection and comprises a variety of neurological disorders, including AIDS dementia complex, HIV-associated encephalopathy and AIDS-associated cognitive decline.

While HIV has not been found to be associated with Alzheimer's disease, HIV-infected brains exhibit defects in the areas affected in AD, particularly the presence of diffuse, largely non-neuritic amyloid plaques in HAND patients with APOE-ε4, as well as atrophy of neurons and neuronal loss in the frontal and temporal cortices (Harris and Harris 2018). Studies also show that patients with HAND and patients with AD both have common misregulated gene expression profiles, indicating altered neuroimmune response along with progressive deficits in synaptic transmission. In addition, it has been found that amyloid beta 42 peptides appear to enhance HIV attachment to facilitate entry into the cells of the central nervous system (Hill et al. 2014).

## The Gut Virome

The gut microbiota plays a key role in the development and functions of the gastrointestinal and immune systems, and perturbations cause disruptions resulting in dysbiosis, increased intestinal permeability, and damage to the intestinal lining, which leads to leaky gut syndrome. Besides archaea, bacteria, fungi and protozoa, the gut has an abundance of viruses, viroids, and eukaryotic and prokaryotic bacteriophages (phages).

Imbalances in the gut microbiota can be caused by phages, and a number of intestinal viruses can move through a defective epithelial lining and enter the central nervous system. Viroids are minimalist plant pathogens that consist of a viroid-specific form of ssRNA (positive single-strand virus) that is very similar to miRNAs (small, non-coding RNAs involved in the regulation of post-translational gene expression) in their ability to spread disease. Because miRNA dysregulation is strongly linked to AD, researchers are studying plant viroids to determine their role in spreading system degenerative disease (Hill et al. 2014).

Common intestinal viruses include *Enterovirus, Norovirus* (Norwalk virus), and *Rotavirus*, which can all cause gastroenteritis, as well as *Adenovirus*, which causes respiratory infections (including the common cold) and conjunctivitis. Viruses that inhabit the small bowel and colon include *Astrovirus*, *Calicivirus*, *Norovirus*, hepatitis E virus, *Coronavirus*, *Torovirus*, and *Adenovirus* (serotypes 40 and 41). *Microviridae* family members found in human gut bacteria include *Microvirus*, *Gokushovirinae*, *Alpavirinae*, and *Picovirinae*. Prophages found in human fecal specimens include *Myoviridae*, *Siphoviridae*, *Podoviridae*, *Tectiviridae*, *Liviviridae*, and *Inoviridae* (Scarpellini et al. 2015).

Besides their ability to disrupt the microbiota, intestinal viruses can cause changes in microbial pathogen-associated molecular patterns, which include gram-negative lipopolysaccharides released from bacterial membranes. As endotoxins, lipopolysaccharides can cause fever and other symptoms.

Bacteriophages are the most prominent members of the gut microbiota, and they outnumber bacteria more than ten-fold. As part of the gut virome, bacteriophages represent 90 percent of the gut viruses. Because bacteriophages can eliminate specific strains of bacteria, they have control over the gastrointestinal microbiota. For instance, the Lak phage infects *Prevotella* species. A gut microbiota rich in Lak will have a low concentration of *Prevotella* species, which, in turn, affects mood, food cravings, and other parameters. A microbiota rich in Lak can also affect intestinal permeability due to its absorption of bacterial antigens (Devoto et al. 2019). The bacterial antigens, in turn, result in an increased number of endotoxins, increased inflammation and dysregulation of the inflammatory response. Bacteriophages are also associated with the formation of prion proteins, which are associated with disruptions in the folding of amyloid protein, a condition linked to neurodegenerative diseases, including Alzheimer's disease. The potential role of bacteriophages in Alzheimer's disease is described in Chapter Twelve.

## Prions

Prions are abnormal acellular (without a cell form) microbes with the ability to cause irregular folding of prion proteins. First found in Creutzfeldt-Jakob disease in humans, the word *prion* (derived from the early term *proteinaceous infectious particle*) was coined in 1982 to distinguish it from other infectious agents. Thus, the word *prion* refers to its composition of an abnormally formed infectious protein with no associated nucleic acids, rendering it distinct from viruses and bacteria.

An important characteristic of prions is their ability to self-propagate. In doing so, prions transform from one conformational state to another, which leads to the creation of new prions (Tetz and Tetz 2017).

Prion proteins are normally found in human cell membranes, although their function is not well understood, and in disease states their shape is altered. Prions are primarily found in the brains of humans, yeast, cattle, deer, elk, and sheep. Although the highest concentrations of prion are found in the central nervous system, high amounts of prion protein are found in the gastrointestinal tract and the enteric nervous system (including the ganglia of the parasympathetic and sympathetic nerves that supply the gastrointestinal tract), as well as the spleen, heart, thymus gland and testes (Davies et al. 2006). While its functions remain unknown, prion protein is thought to regulate synaptic function in neurons, possibly by regulating copper metabolism. It's also been suggested that prion protein may protect neurons in response to stimuli such as oxidative stress (Davies et al. 2006).

When prions, which are transmissible, lead to abnormal folding of the prion protein, an infectious isoform is produced, which is known as $PrP^{sc}$. This abnormal isoform, when transmitted to animals, leads to memory and personality changes, depression, unsteady gait, slurred speech, tremors, insomnia, and confusion. Prions cause diseases known as transmissible spongiform encephalopathies (TSEs). TSEs progress over time and culminate in conditions of fatal brain damage.

These diseases are characterized by numerous small holes in the cortex, which cause this area of the brain, when viewed microscopically, to have the structure of a sponge. While prions are primarily transmitted through contaminated food or transplant organs, in yeast, transmission involves the passing of a genetic trait from mother to daughter cells in cytoplasm rather than through a cell nucleus.

In animals, TSEs include scrapie in sheep; bovine spongiform encephalopathy (BSE), which is also known as mad cow's disease, in cattle; and chronic wasting disease (CWD) in deer and elk.

## Creutzfeldt-Jakob Disease

TSEs found to occur in humans include Creutzfeldt-Jakob disease (CJD), which has three subtypes: sporadic CJD, hereditary or familiar CJD, and acquired CJD, which includes both iatrogenic and variant CJD, which are caused by exposure to bovine prions; Gerstmann- Sträussler–Scheinker syndrome (GSS); fatal familial insomnia; kuru, which was identified in the Fore tribe of Papua New Guinea; and variably protease-sensitive prionopathy. These diseases can be difficult to distinguish from one another because of their overlapping signs and symptoms, although the rate of disease progression offers clues. Classic or sporadic CJD progresses over months, whereas the variant form progresses over a period of years.

Researchers have found that kuru was initially transmitted during a funeral in which the brain of a dead tribe member was removed, cooked and eaten. In experiments, brain extracts from individuals who died from kuru or CJD have been injected into the brains of chimpanzees to confirm that this form of transmission effectively causes TSE disease development.

Most TSEs are due to the ingestion or inoculation of substances infected with infective prions. Pathology in all forms of orally acquired TSEs occurs when the host's encoded prion protein takes on the conformation of its infectious misfolded counterpart, PrP$^{sc}$. Patients have also inadvertently developed CJD after receiving human growth hormone therapy and corneal transplants. In addition, some forms of CJD have been inherited in children of infected parents. Familial CJD and fatal familial insomnia can also arise from the prion gene as a consequence of germline mutations and possibly somatic mutations—for instance, in sporadic cases of CJD (Davies et al. 2006).

While memory loss and unsteady gait occur early in the course of the disease, overt symptoms—such as chorea (abnormal movement disorder, a type of dyskinesis), dystonia (a movement disorder in which muscles spontaneously contract, causing the affected body part to twist involuntarily, causing repetitive movements or abnormal postures), myoclonus (jerking movements), and dementia—occur later.

Prion protein amyloid plaques have been found in brain samples from patients diagnosed with TSEs, including CJD, GSS, kuru and the animal prion disease scrapie. CJD is also known to coexist with AD, causing a condition of mixed CJD/AD, which has been found to occur in 2–15 percent of studies using brain bank specimens (Harris and Harris 2018).

## Prions and Alzheimer's Disease

Genes regulating prion formation reside in the prion-forming domain (PFD), which is characterized by disordered, long, minimally complex proteins. Amyloid cores are found in several of these PFDs and also in certain yeast prions. In diseases associated with protein misfolding and its aggregates, such as Parkinson's disease and Alzheimer's disease, certain soluble proteins are converted into amyloid fibrils.

Researchers have found that amyloid beta oligomer regulates the interaction between intracellular protein mediators and the synaptic receptor complex that is composed of cellular prion protein (PrP$^C$) and the metatrobic glutamate receptor 5 (mGluR5). In addition, this oligomer on the prion-receptor complex affects glutamate activation. The disruption of normal signaling cascades caused by oligomers contributes to neurodegeneration and dementia (Haas and Strittmatter 2016).

In a related genome-wide expression cloning experiment conducted in 2009, cellular prion protein was identified as a cell surface-binding site for amyloid beta oligomers. These oligomers bind to cellular prion protein with high affinity, and the role of cellular prion protein in Alzheimer's disease is well established. Altered function and loss of excitatory synapses is an early step in the brain dysfunction exhibited in Alzheimer's disease. Mice bred to develop AD-related phenotypes can be prevented from developing dementia by blocking either the cellular prion protein or the mGluR5.

Because mGluR5 physically and genetically couples PrP$^C$ to intracellular signaling proteins during acute exposure to amyloid beta oligomers, interfering with enzymes such as the kinases (which mediate this process) can prevent this coupling, thereby preventing disease development. While more studies on the role of prions in Alzheimer's disease are needed, they appear to play a role by interfering with excitatory signaling (Haas and Strittmatter 2016).

It's thought that infectious prions follow the same route as other infectious agents from the gastrointestinal tract to the central nervous system with the aid of the immune system. The lymphatic system is also believed to serve as a route to the central nervous system because of the role of the spleen in harboring infectious prions.

Some of the most studied endogenous prions are the amyloid proteins, which increase in response to infection. Prion proteins are also found to be present in bacteriophages, bacteria and archaea.

## Summary

Although the *Herpes simplex* viruses, *Herpes zoster*, and the human herpes viruses 6 and 7 appear to have the strongest association with Alzheimer's disease development, other viruses have also been implicated, including cytomegalovirus, Epstein-Barr virus, and the hepatitis C virus. In addition, bacteriophages influence disease development through their effects on the microbiome, and prion proteins also play a role. Although infectious prions are a well-known cause of dementia in individuals infected with TSEs, these proteins have an effect on signaling molecules and the development of neurodegeneration in individuals with Alzheimer's disease.

# EIGHT

# Bacterial Infections

Postmortem studies conducted on the brains of patients who died from Alzheimer's disease routinely show a seven-fold increase in microbes, along with a wider variety of bacterial species when compared to age-matched subjects without cognitive impairment. James Hill and colleagues, in their 2014 article "Pathogenic Microbes, the Microbiome, and Alzheimer's Disease," write, "Virtually every type of microbe known has been implicated in contributing to the susceptibility and pathogenesis of the AD process."

A wide array of pathogenic microorganisms has been implicated in AD. This is not surprising since most bacteria finding their way into the brain originate in the oral cavity, the lungs, and the gastrointestinal and urinary tracts. Conditions of delirium, which are often caused by infection, correlated with an eight-fold increase in dementia development, and cognition in AD subjects worsened after an episode of delirium. The presence of numerous infections over a 4-year period has been found to double the risk of dementia, and cognitive decline has been observed within two to six months of a resolved infection, presumably due to the continued presence of pro-inflammatory cytokines (McManus and Heneka 2017). Vaccination against influenza has been shown to reduce the risk of AD development, and antibiotic treatment has been observed to slow cognitive decline in patients with known infections.

It's also been noted that certain non-cognitive symptoms often seen in patients with AD, such as agitation, aggression, and psychosis, can be triggered by an infection arising almost anywhere in the body. Humans infected with rabies, for instance, are known to become aggressive and bite other humans. Some bacteria appear to play a more prominent role in Alzheimer's than others, and these bacteria are the focus of this chapter.

## Association with the Gut Microbiome and APOE-ε4

Most neurological disorders are known to have a progressive, age-related, and geographical character. For instance, the incidence of AD varies a great deal in different human populations and is influenced by diet, biological environment, the complexity of the gut microbiome, and one's exposure to microbes (Hill et al. 2014).

The countries most affected by Alzheimer's include (listed in the order of the highest rate) Finland, the United States, Canada, Iceland, Sweden, Switzerland, Norway, Denmark, Netherlands, and Belgium. Those with the lowest rates include India, Cambodia, Georgia, and Singapore (Hillis 2015). The United States has the second highest incidence of AD globally, and the state with the highest incidence of AD is Alaska.

While the turmeric (curcumin) widely used in India is said to offer protection because of its high antioxidant content, the countries with the lowest incidence of AD rarely consume processed foods. Japanese people living in their native country have a low incidence of AD, but when they move to the United States and adopt a Western diet, their incidence of AD rises.

The presence of the APOE-ε4 allele is a risk factor for developing AD. In postmortem studies, the brains of individuals with the APOE-ε4 allele are more likely to show the presence of pathogenic microbes. The combined risk factors of infection and the presence of the APOE-ε4 allele are thought to play a major role in AD development.

Bacterial infection in the central nervous system can be transmitted via the nerves and lymph vessels that connect it to the oronasal cavity and the gastrointestinal tract. Both the gastrointestinal lining (epithelial barrier) and the blood-brain barrier become more permeable with age, facilitating the entry of microbes and their neurotoxins. Besides aging, chronic bacterial or viral infections can also progressively alter the blood-brain barrier permeability.

# Mycobacterium

*Mycobacterium tuberculosis* (*M. tuberculosis*), the cause of tuberculosis, is a member of the Class *Actinobacteria*. *M. tuberculosis* has been known to cause both dementia and amyloid plaques since 1769, when the Scottish physician Robert Whytt described 20 cases of dementia caused by tuberculosis (Broxmeyer 2016, 66). It was also established by 1860 that these brain plaques could occur in any type of tuberculosis, whether the brain had been infected or not.

When Alois Alzheimer described dementia in his patient Auguste Deter, he strayed from the term *senile dementia* coined by Oskar Fischer ten years earlier, instead calling his "new" disease "presenile" dementia (and later Alzheimer's disease) since Deter was only in her early 50s when she was institutionalized. In cases where dementia, like Deter's, is associated with tuberculosis, the infectious agent, *M. tuberculosis*, is reported to have first infected the patient early in life (usually during childhood) and then remained, causing a chronic attack on the immune system. The amyloid plaques in Deter's and other cases of tuberculosis-related meningoencephalitis show evidence of the filamentous bacilli (or Drüsen) described by Fischer. In 1910, tuberculosis was one of the leading causes of death from infection globally. Worldwide, in 2018 tuberculosis was reported to be one of the top ten leading causes of death and the leading cause of death from a single infectious agent (World Health Organization 2019, 18).

## *Mycobacterium* Species

*Mycobacterium* is a genus of *Actinobacteria*, with its own family, the *Mycobacteriaceae*. *Mycobacteriaceae* contains more than 190 different species, with the most common being *Mycobacterium tuberculosis*. A review of the medical literature shows numerous cases of meningoencephalitis caused by tuberculosis initially confused with Alzheimer's disease. With appropriate treatment, dementia in these cases was resolved. It's not surprising that the antibiotic rifampicin—widely used to treat *Mycobacterium* infections—is listed in a review of agents that have been found to have beneficial effects in Alzheimer's disease (Appleby et al. 2013). The preventive effect of rifampicin on Alzheimer's disease has also been reported in Japan, using a dose of 450 mg daily for one year in patients with *Mycobacterium* infection and AD-type hypometabolism (Iizuka et al. 2017).

Dementia is associated with other species besides *M. tuberculosis*. In 2004, researchers at the University of Toronto described a case of rapidly progressive dementia caused by *Mycobacterium neoaurum* meningoencephalitis (Heckman et al. 2004; Geschwind et al. 2007). Non-tuberculosis *Mycobacterial* infection, associated with a productive cough and chronic obstructive pulmonary disease, is known to be more common in elderly subjects, especially slender women. These pathogens are found in soil, tap water, showerheads, steam from hot tubs, and soil from parks and gardens, and they are often present in biofilms. Commonly found in pulmonary conditions, these pathogens are also common in subjects with dementia.

# Chlamydia pneumoniae

*Chlamydia pneumoniae* (*Chlamydophila pneumoniae*; *C. pneumoniae*), an obligate gram-negative intracellular bacterium, and a common cause of respiratory diseases (including pneumonia), is the microorganism considered by many to be the most plausible candidate as a bacterial cause of AD (Sochocka et al. 2017). Its initial entry into the body typically occurs through the mouth or nose, and it is known to thrive on mucosal surfaces. *C. pneumoniae* is also associated with coronary artery disease, arthritis, multiple sclerosis, and meningoencephalitis (Balin et al. 1998; Hill et al. 2014).

In one 1998 study, atypical extracellular *C. pneumoniae* antigens were found in the neocortex, senile plaques, and neurofibrillary tangles of the brain in 90 percent of AD subjects and in 5 percent of control subjects. This organism has also been identified in neurons in the brains of AD subjects (Sochocka et al. 2017). In addition, signs of neuroinflammation were present (Balin et al. 1998). In a more recent study, Brian Balin and his team identified *C. pneumoniae* infection in microglia and astroglia in the brains of AD patients, suggesting that inflammation initiated by infected cells might be involved in the disease process (Balin et al. 2018). For the past twenty years, Balin, a world-renowned AD researcher, has studied the role of *C. pneumoniae* in late-onset AD (LOAD), and he sees the need for clinical trials.

*C. pneumoniae* has a two-phased developmental cycle and depends on energy and nutrients in the form of sphingomyelin and cholesterol, which are gathered from its host. The first phase of development involves the infectious extracellular form of *C. pneumoniae*, which is known as the elementary body. The elementary body primarily infects epithelial cells, but it also infects the astroglia, microglia, and neurons of the central nervous system.

As a final step in development, the elementary body reorganizes into a reticulate body, which is the metabolically active form of the organism, able to undergo multiple cycles of cell division and replication. This process yields the infectious elementary body causing chronic infection. *C. pneumoniae* is able to take up residence in monocytes, causing long-term infection while it is in a state known as persistence. Similar to other *Chlamydia* species, *C. pneumoniae* is viable and metabolically active but refrains from completing its developmental cycle. Persistent chlamydial infection is resistant to antibiotic treatment.

In a comparison of the characteristics of AD and those of *C. pneumoniae* infection, it's found that every aspect of AD can be explained by this infection. For instance, the calcium dysregulation in AD can be linked to the increased influx of calcium in *C. pneumoniae* infection. The imbalance in the neurotransmitter kynurenine and quinolinic acid can be linked to *C. pneumoniae*'s activation of interferon gamma, which causes an increase in the damaging quinolinic acid. The iron dysregulation seen in AD can be related to the iron deposits in *C. pneumoniae* infection that lead to free (unliganded) iron. The leakage of the blood-brain barrier in AD can be linked to the increased barrier permeability caused by this infection (Fülöp et al. 2018, "Role of Microbes").

Since Balin's early studies, numerous other studies have confirmed the presence of *C. pneumoniae* in the brains of individuals with AD. In one of Balin's recent publications, he and his colleagues explain that the entorhinal cortex and the hippocampal formation, both olfactory structures, show the earliest signs of damage in LOAD. He notes that *C. pneumoniae* has been identified in both human and animal olfactory bulbs. In animals, the microbes appear to spread from the olfactory bulbs into the brain proper (Balin et al. 2018). An early symptom that occurs in both mild cognitive impairment and AD is an impairment of the sense of smell (olfactory dysfunction). In addition, because respiratory failure and pneumonia are common causes of death in patients with AD, a causative effect from *C. pneumoniae* is the subject of intense investigation.

## Spirochetes

Spirochetes, as their name suggests, are long, slender, tightly coiled motile gram-negative bacteria with axial filaments, which resemble bacterial flagella. With the exception of *Treponema*, these filaments reside within an outer sheath that runs along the outside of the protoplasm. These filaments allow the bacterium to move and rotate. Aerobic and anaerobic (living in oxygen-free environments) forms of *Treponema* exist. Spirochetes are most often found in liquids, such as mud, water, blood, and lymph fluid.

Infectious diseases caused by spirochetes include syphilis, which is caused by *Treponema pallidum*; yaws, caused by *Treponema pertenue*; Lyme disease, caused by *Borrelia burgdorferi*; relapsing fever, caused by *Borrelia recurrentis*; gingivitis and periodontitis, caused by oral treponemes; and leptospirosis, which is caused by *Leptospira* and primarily infects wild mammals, although it may be a secondary infection in humans.

The late stage of syphilis, which emerged in the late fifteenth century, is characterized by dementia, indicating that spirochetal infection can cause a type of dementia with features very similar to those seen in AD. First discovered as the causative agent of syphilis by Fritz Schaudinn and Erich Hoffman in 1905, the pale-colored *Treponema pallidum* survived despite toxic treatments such as mercury and arsenic, which harmed those afflicted more than it harmed the spirochetes (Quetel 1990, 4).

All of the features used to diagnose AD are seen in syphilis, including amyloid beta (Aβ) deposits, the presence of spirochetal colonies indistinguishable from curli fibers, and senile plaques. Each curli fiber in AD corresponds to a single spirochete in syphilis, and each senile plaque in AD resembles a spirochetal colony (Miklossy 2017).

In addition, Judith Miklossy, MD, has detected the presence of spirochetes (primarily oral treponemes) in 100 percent of the patients she studied who died from AD; these microorganisms were absent in control subjects. In confirmed AD patients who were living, Miklossy and her team found spirochetes in the brain, blood and spinal fluid. Spirochetes in moderate numbers were also found in patients in the preclinical stages of AD. Miklossy reports that other authors have detected *Borrelia burgdorferi* in the brains of AD patients 14 times more frequently than in controls, and they found oral treponemes in more than 90 percent of AD patients (Miklossy 2017).

Miklossy writes that because of their curly shape, spirochetes are a logical candidate for infection in the brain. Treponemes, in particular, have a great affinity for neurons, and there are many spirochetes residing in the human body. As is the case with syphilis, spirochetes frequently co-infect their hosts with other fungi and viruses, usually HSV-1, microorganisms frequently encountered in patients with AD.

## Neuroborreliosis in Lyme Disease

Because spirochetes are found in the brain of individuals with AD, it was once suspected that Lyme disease could lead to AD. Fortunately, this isn't the case, although infection with *Borrelia burgdorferi* can lead to several forms of dementia, with the most severe disease being Lyme neuroborreliosis, which is easily distinguished from Lyme encephalopathy or post–Lyme syndrome. In neuroborreliosis, an examination of cerebrospinal fluid shows *Borrelia burgdorferi* antibodies along with elevated concentrations of protein.

The development of dementia is rapid in neuroborreliosis, occurring within two months to two years after a tick bite. Gait disturbances are one of the first manifestations, followed by impaired cognitive function. In one study of 48 patients, 45 were earlier diagnosed with Bannwarth's syndrome, a well-characterized painful radiculoneuritis (inflammation of one or more roots of the cerebrospinal nerves). Overall, symptoms of neuroborreliosis are manifestations of chronic progressing meningoencephalomyelitis, which responds very well to antibiotic treatment. In this study, even when symptoms of cognitive impairment persisted for as long as one year, antibiotic treatment resulted in improvement in as little as two weeks. The most common treatment was a 2–4 week course of the antibiotic ceftriaxone (Kristoferitsch et al. 2018).

## Oral Gingivitis and Periodontitis

The human oral cavity is rich in commensal microbes that help protect against invasion of undesirable intruders. However, when there is an imbalance of microbial flora, this imbalance or condition of dysbiosis can contribute to both oral and systemic diseases. Common oral diseases include dental caries, periodontitis, gingivitis, and oral mucosal diseases. Systemic diseases include gastrointestinal diseases and diseases of the central nervous system, including Alzheimer's disease.

The oral cavity has several distinct habitats, including the teeth, gingival sulcus, tongue, hard and soft palates, and tonsils. The oral cavity also serves as a tube connecting its exterior entrance to the digestive and respiratory tracts, providing ample access to colonization by foreign microorganisms.

### Oral Microbes

The Human Oral Microbiome Database maintains a listing of 150 genera and 700 species of microbes found in healthy humans. However, obtaining specimens for culture has its own set of problems, making the listing incomplete. The NIH Common Fund Human Microbiome Project was established to provide a comprehensive characterization of human microbiota based on a total of 4,788 specimens from 242 screened and phenotyped healthy adults.

The results of the NIH project showed that age was a determinant. That is, healthy females or males of the same age groups were likely to have similar oral microbiotas. Diet also played a role in that the change from hunter-gatherer to farming populations (based on genome results showing ancestry) led to more pathogenic organisms in the farming group. The oral microbiota was also influenced by breastfeeding in infancy, gender, eating sweets at night, and level of education (Gao et al. 2018).

### Periodontal Diseases

Periodontal diseases can be classified as either gingival diseases or periodontitis. Periodontal disease results in a generalized destruction of the structures that support the teeth, such as the gingiva and the alveolar bone, causing a potential risk for systemic diseases. In a study of patients with generalized chronic, localized aggressive periodontitis, or peri-implantitis, the red complex bacteria (which include *Porphyromonas gingivalis*, *Treponema denticola*, and *Tannerella forsythia*) were the most prevalent, with very high levels in all groups. The red complex bacteria, which also include *Fusobacterium nucleatum*, are recognized as the most important pathogens in adult periodontal disease.

The green and blue complex bacteria were less prevalent in these patients, with the exception of *Aggregatibacter actinomycetemcomitans*, which was detected in all localized aggressive cases of periodontitis. In comparison, healthy adults without periodontal disease had the greatest diversity in their oral microbiotas.

Peri-implantitis refers to the infectious disease that can occur in people with dental implants. It is characterized by inflammation of the surrounding tissues, bleeding of the surrounding tissue when probed, and bone loss. Different oral microbiomes are found in people who develop peri-implantitis when compared to normal individuals. In particular, individuals with peri-implantitis were more likely to have *Eubacterium* (a family of gram-positive, anaerobic bacilli), and several species in this family are considered oral pathogens. Various *Eubacterium* and related species (for instance, *Filifactor alocis*, *Mogibacterium timidum*, *Mogibacterium vescum*, and *Pseudoramibacter alactolyticus*) have been recovered from endodontic, periodontal, and other infectious oral lesions.

## Diseases of the Oral Mucosa

Diseases affecting the oral mucosa include oral leukoplakia, oral lichen planus, and systemic lupus erythematosus. Several studies have demonstrated that bacteria contribute to these mucosal diseases. Dysbiosis of the oral microbiome contributes to inflammatory bowel disease, Alzheimer's disease, diabetes, rheumatoid arthritis and atherosclerosis (Gao et al. 2018).

## Association with Alzheimer's Disease

A number of studies have reported that tooth loss, particularly when it occurs before age 35, is a significant risk factor for AD and dementia. Other studies have also shown increased levels of the cytokines interleukin-1 beta, interleukin-6, and tumor necrosis factor–alpha (TNF-α) in patients with Alzheimer's disease. In one study researchers tested AD subjects and controls for TNF-α and serum antibodies to the oral microbes *Actinobacillus actinomycetemcomitans*, *Tannerella forsythia* and *Porphyromonas gingivalis* (*P. gingivalis*). These three species were identified at the 1996 World Workshop in Periodontics as causally related to periodontics and its progression. These species are also known to cause a specific humoral immune response to the host (Kamer et al. 2010).

Levels of TNF-α and antibodies to these oral bacteria were significantly higher in AD patients compared to controls. The presence of oral treponemes such as *Treponema denticola* (*T. denticola*) has also been found to be higher in the brains of AD subjects compared to control subjects (Kamer et al. 2010).

In a study conducted at the University of Kentucky, subjects had normal cognitive function at baseline testing of bacterial antibody levels. At the ten-year follow-up, patients who showed cognitive defects had increased antibody levels of the oral anaerobes *Fusobacterium nucleatum* (*F. nucleatum*) and *Prevotella intermedia* (Gao et al. 2018).

    *F. nucleatum* is one of the most abundant bacterial species found in the oral cavities of both diseased and healthy dental patients. It is associated with a number of periodontal diseases ranging from mild treatable gingivitis to advanced irreversible forms of periodontitis. It is also frequently associated with endodontic infections. The prevalence of *F. nucleatum* increases with disease, severity, pocket depth and the degree of inflammation.

## *P. gingivalis* and Oral Treponemes

    Most studies of oral microbes and AD have focused on *P. gingivalis* and the oral treponemes. In studies, *P. gingivalis* has been found in 96 percent of the brains of AD patients, and *P. gingivalis* DNA has also been identified in the cerebrospinal fluid of living AD patients (Gao et al. 2018; Dominy et al. 2019). Neurotoxic arginine or lysine-specific protease enzymes called gingipains (also known as RgpA, RgpB and Kgp) are involved in the adherence to and infection of epithelial cells and neurons, destruction of red blood cells, disruption and manipulation of the inflammatory response, and the degradation of host proteins and tissues.

    In AD, *P. gingivalis* is known to disrupt the blood-brain barrier (BBB) and promote deposits of amyloid beta protein. Studies of the AD brain show that gingipains have been found in the neurons of the dentate nucleus in the hippocampus. In addition, gingipains have detrimental effects on tau, a protein needed for normal neuronal function, and they have been found to target APOE protein, which could generate neurotoxic APOE fragments in the brain. The APOE-ε4 gene is more susceptible to *P. gingivalis* because of its greater abundance of argine residues than the other alleles (Dominy et al. 2019).

    When secreted by *P. gingivalis*, gingipains are transported to the outer bacterial membrane surfaces and partially released in soluble and outer membrane vesicle associated forms. Because *P. gingivalis* is difficult to eradicate with broad-spectrum antibiotics, researchers have designed a way to block the neurotoxic gingipains by using Kgp inhibitors that stop their proteolytic activity, which reduces their virulence. Kgp, which removes nutrient hemoglobin from red blood cells, is essential for the survival of *P. gingivalis* because it generates peptide nutrients essential for the bacteria's growth. Stephen Dominy and his team have completed Phase I trials with the drug CORE-388, which is Cortexyme's lead compound and gingipain inhibitor.

It was tested for safety in healthy older adults and patients with Alzheimer's disease, and it was very well tolerated.

As of late 2019, Dominy and his team are moving into a larger, Phase II clinical trial to test the efficacy of the drug; if successful, it will be a new treatment for Alzheimer's disease. More information on the trial (NCT03823404) can be found at clinicaltrials.gov (Dominy et al. 2019).

## Protein Markers

Many studies involving AD have striven to find biological markers to help diagnose AD. A 2007 landmark study identified 18 plasma proteins that could predict the development of AD. The results were confirmed and showed high sensitivity and specificity. TNF-α and several other immune system proteins were among the protein markers used to predict AD. Angela Kamer and her team at the Dental School at New York University found that these markers, as well as the antibodies to the oral pathogens studied, were shown to accurately predict AD (Kamer et al. 2010).

Bacterial colonies increase in strength when they unite with the proteins, polyuronic and nucleic acids, and lipids that they release to form biofilms. The bacterial species in biofilms are difficult to culture and identify because they need other species to attach to for their survival. Researchers in the United Kingdom have found that when removed from their preferred oral environment, the oral biofilms in aged individuals may migrate to other parts of the body. In immunosenescence, the aged immune system is no longer as vigilant (Shoemark and Allen 2015).

Among the many oral bacteria found in the AD brain, the most prevalent class has been found to be the oral spirochetes. Both AD subjects and controls showed the presence of treponemes in the brain and trigeminal ganglia, but *Treponema maltophilum* was only found in the AD brain. This is similar to the finding that lipopolysaccharide released from *P. gingivalis* is found in the brains of AD brains but not in those of control subjects (Shoemark and Allen 2015).

The APOE-ε4 gene is highly correlated with the risk of late-onset AD, with an odds ratio of 12.9 for homozygous ε4 carriers compared to ε4/ε3 heterozygote carriers. APOE-ε4 is known to compromise the integrity of the BBB by activating the cyclophilin A matrix metalloproteinase MP-9 pathways, facilitating the entry of microbes across the BBB. The trigeminal and olfactory nerves also connect directly from the oronasal cavity to the brain, providing another route for oral microbes to enter the brain.

## Oral Considerations

The results of studies conducted in the past two decades clearly show as much as a seven-fold increase in pathogenic oral microbes in the brains of AD patients compared to the brains of control subjects. The AD subjects, with an average age in the mid–80s, were born in the 1920s or thereabouts. Dentistry was a different field at this time, and several factors need to be taken into consideration.

The sterility and precision of dental equipment has improved over the years, but even in the 1950s it was primitive compared to that used today. While tooth loss is now linked to dementia, in the past patients often waited to see a dentist until a tooth was beyond repair. Dentures were considered a quick fix, and it wasn't until the 1960s that the concept of saving teeth emerged. When a root canal was required, it was performed immediately, whereas today patients are often first treated with antibiotics.

Nitrous oxide was widely used until around 1990 and is still in use, although now patients with compromised immune systems are warned against its use. More recently, nitrous oxide–induced neurotoxicity has been implicated in the development of long-lasting cognitive defects when administered at either age extreme (Sanders et al. 2008).

Xylocaine, used as a local anesthetic in dentistry, is a combination of lidocaine and epinephrine, which is used to facilitate the movement of lidocaine through tissues. Studies regarding the ability of epinephrine to help with the migration of microbes from the oral cavity are needed to gain a better understanding of the ways in which pathogenic microbes make their way into the brain. The practices in dentistry, primarily older techniques, may differ from the clinical picture in dentistry today and should be correlated with modern studies of the oral microbiome. The associations of mercury and fluoride in AD are described in Chapter Ten.

## Other Bacterial Associations with AD

In studies of bacterial infection in the brains of AD subjects, *Proteobacteria* was the most prominent in both AD patients and in control subjects. The phylum of *Proteobacteria* includes *Escherichia* species such as *Escherichia coli* (*E. coli*), *Salmonella*, *Vibrio*, *Helicobacter*, *Yersinia*, *Legionellales* and others. After *Proteobacteria*, the most abundant bacteria were *Firmicutes*, *Actinobacteria* and *Bacteroides*, which are also abundant gut microbes. At the family level, *Burkholderiaceae* and *Staphylococcaceae* were seen in higher percentages in the AD brains than in control brains (Alonso et al. 2018).

*Helicobacter pylori* (*H. pylori*) and *Proprionibacterium acnes* (*P. acnes*) have also been found to be associated with AD and, because of their role in chronic inflammation, may play a more significant role than other species found in the brains of AD patients. *H. pylori* is a gram-negative gut microbe. The presence of antibodies to *H. pylori* in older individuals is associated with decreased cognitive function. Research also shows that AD patients have an increased rate of positive *H. pylori* antibody results in both serum and cerebrospinal fluid. Individuals with AD are likewise reported to have an increased incidence of *H. pylori* infection of the gastric mucosa (cause of gastric ulcers) compared to control subjects. Among AD patients, subjects infected with *H. pylori* had more severe dementia and increased levels of tau and pro-inflammatory cytokines in their spinal fluid. In addition, patients with AD and infection who received treatment and remained free of *H. pylori* for two years showed improved cognitive function, whereas patients who did not respond to treatment and were still infected had worse cognitive function (McManus and Heneka 2017).

While *P. acnes* is primarily found on the skin, in a small study this microbe was found to be present in the brains of AD patients with a distribution ten-fold higher than that of *Proteobacteria*. *P. acnes* has been found to be associated with implants, and it persists in circulating macrophages, which may explain its route to the brain.

## Bacterial Endotoxins and Iron

Besides the effects of bacterial infection, gram-negative bacteria contain lipopolysaccharide molecules that may play a role in causing sporadic AD. Lipopolysaccharide molecules are endotoxins, and the blood levels of lipopolysaccharides in AD patients are three times as high as the levels in control subjects.

In addition, gram-negative bacterial lipopolysaccharide molecules have been found in the brains of AD subjects and control subjects, with much higher levels seen in AD brains. These lipopolysaccharides have been found in amyloid plaques as well as neurons and oligodendrocytes in AD brains. In oligodendrocytes, the presence of lipopolysaccharides results in signs of injury and degraded myelin basic protein. Researchers have proposed that bacterial lipopolysaccharides act on the toll-like receptor 4 (TLR-4) of immune system cells to cause the production of pro-inflammatory cytokines that increase amyloid beta protein levels and to produce the myelin injury seen in AD (Zhan et al. 2018). A number of studies have found that lipopolysaccharides can lead to neuroinflammation and drive amyloid beta formation (Pretorius et al. 2016).

### Iron Dysregulation in AD

Etheresia Pretorius and her team in South Africa have been examining the causes of the excessive neuroinflammation seen in the AD brain. Their findings support the theory that in AD the neuroinflammation is most likely the result of a systemic inflammatory condition. They've found that all the factors (such as the expression of pro-inflammatory cytokines; the pathological loss of neurons, astrocytes, and microglia; and the increased presence of reactive oxygen species seen in AD, Parkinson's disease, multiple sclerosis, amyotrophic lateral sclerosis, and Huntington's disease) can be attributed to iron dysregulation. In AD, iron dysregulation is a well-known symptom characterized by increased iron inside amyloid beta deposits, increased levels of ferritin in the AD brain, and increased blood levels of free iron. This situation may explain the success of chelation therapies used in AD that reduce cognitive function (Pretorius et al. 2016; Hopperton et al. 2018).

Iron is stored in the brain as either heavy or light subunits. Ferritin is a blood cell protein that stores iron. While neurons and other cells primarily contain heavy ferritin (the least reactive form), glial cells contain the light subunit, which can generate free radicals during the inflammatory response. For this reason, ferritin is considered an acute-phase reactant, and high serum levels are indicators of inflammation, particularly increases in microglial cell number and activation. Higher numbers of ferritin-positive microglia cells were found in the amygdala, entorhinal cortex, and frontal, occipital, parietal and temporal neocortices of the AD brain when compared to those of control subjects (Hopperton et al. 2018).

Whereas viruses can remain latent in human cells, bacteria and archaea can stop growing and replicating while still existing in a dormant state, called a state of persistence. The excess iron in AD is thought to bring these microorganisms out of their dormant state, allowing them to become infectious, so that they, in turn, cause neuroinflammation and cause the production of amyloid beta protein.

## Summary

Brain concentrations of various bacterial species are seven-fold higher in patients with AD than seen in control subjects. In studies of the AD brain, *C. pneumoniae*, spirochetes, *H. pylori*, and several pathogenic oral microbes are the bacterial species most often seen. Treatments that eradicate the causative bacteria lead to improvement in cognition in living patients diagnosed with AD. A novel treatment for inhibiting gingipains released from *P. gingivalis* showed good results in Phase I clinical trials, with Phase II trials scheduled for late 2019.

Infection itself isn't the only causative factor in AD. Lipopolysaccharides released from the membranes of gram-negative bacteria also contribute to pathology in AD, primarily by inducing neuroinflammation and driving amyloid beta protein production. The iron dysregulation commonly seen in AD is thought to activate dormant bacteria in the brain, causing persistent infection, as well as neuroinflammation, and contributing to the disease process in AD.

# NINE

# Fungal and Protozoan Infections

Besides the many bacteria, viruses, and bacteriophages that make up the human microbiota, a number of fungi normally inhabit the human body. While our relationship with fungi can be one of commensalism, with one party benefiting and the other unaffected or neutral, fungi can also function as parasites (organisms that live on or inside a living host at the expense of the host). The parasites found to be highly associated with Alzheimer's disease include several varieties of yeast and the protozoan parasite *Toxoplasmosis gondii*.

## The Mycobiome in Health and Disease

Mycology is the scientific study of fungi, and the mycobiome represents the genetic material from all the fungi on one's skin and inside an individual's body. Fungi include yeasts, molds, and mushrooms. Yeasts and molds are usually commensal microbes, helping create a balanced microbiome in humans and alerting us when food has gone bad. However, when we ingest certain molds or yeasts, particularly *Candida* species, we develop fungal overgrowth (often from the use of antibiotics), and infection develops.

Fungi are eukaryotes and have no plant properties. Fungal walls contain a polysaccharide called chitin, which is not found in any other microbes. The presence of chitin, the fungal proteins 1,3-beta-glucan and beta-tubulin, the fungal enzymes enolase or chitinase, or other fungal elements inside the body is an indication of fungal infection. These elements have been found in the blood, brain, and blood vessels of individuals with AD, suggesting that fungal infections may contribute to AD development or increase its risk.

A number of reports over the past five years have described fungal infections as contributors to the progression of AD. Studies have also shown that the parts of the brain infected with fungi correspond with the parts of the brain affected in Alzheimer's disease. Many different fungal species have been detected in the AD brain, including *Saccharomyces cerevisiae* (*S. cerevisiae*), *Malassezia globosa* (*M. globosa*), *Malassezia restricta* (*M. restricta*), and *Penicillium*. Cerebrospinal fluid (CSF) analysis of AD patients showed the presence of DNA from *S. cerevisiae*, *M. globosa*, and *M. restricta* (McManus and Heneka 2017). In addition, CSF levels of *Candida albicans* (*C. albicans*) and *Candida glabrata* (*C. glabrata*) proteins were significantly greater in AD patients than in control subjects. It was also observed that many AD patients showed DNA evidence of co-infection with multiple fungal species, while no evidence of fungal DNA was observed in control samples (McManus and Heneka 2017).

It should be noted that prior to the development of antibody binding tests and DNA analyses, it was assumed that the central nervous system and vascular system were completely sterile. It's now known that traces and small amounts of microbes are occasionally found in these bodily systems, particularly in elderly subjects (including those with good cognitive function).

## Candida Species

Fungi belong to the Kingdom Fungi, and their classification in a particular phylum depends on their mode of reproduction. Fungal cells can reproduce by budding, through hyphal extension or by forming spores. Fungal spores can reproduce sexually via the fusion of two gametes or asexually as transported spores.

Yeasts are single-celled eukaryote microorganisms and classified in the Kingdom Fungi. Because yeasts are evolutionarily diverse, they are classified into two separate phyla, *Ascomycota* (or sac fungi) and *Basidiomycota* (or higher fungi), which together constitute the subkingdom *Dikarya*. Yeasts produce colonies that are similar to bacterial colonies and can easily become enmeshed within biofilms containing several microorganisms. Unlike bacteria, yeasts and other fungi do not secrete toxins. Tissue damage in fungal infections is due to direct invasion of tissue. Yeasts differ from most other fungi, which exclusively grow as thread-like hyphae (filament-like projections that extend from the fungal cell). While many fungi have cytoplasm contained within the hyphae that's not divided into cells, some fungi have septate hyphae, which means the cytoplasm within the hypha is divided into cells by cross walls or septa. Hyphae can easily intertwine to form a mass called a mycelium or thallus that becomes more resistant to treatment.

Some fungi can alternate between a yeast phase and a hyphal phase, depending on environmental conditions. Such fungi are termed dimorphic (having two distinct shapes) and can be very pathogenic. *C. albicans* and *S. cerevisiae* are dimorphic fungi.

Although it normally lives harmlessly on the skin and mucous membranes of the mouth, gastrointestinal tract and genitourinary tract, *C. albicans* is an opportunistic yeast. When the opportunity arises for it to dominate, it flourishes, growing rapidly and leading to fungal infections (mycoses) of the mouth, skin, and vagina. This usually happens when multiple predisposing factors cause the yeast population to multiply, escaping the normal patrol by resident bacteria, which keep the yeast population in check. In opportunistic infections, the yeast cells sprout a hyphal outgrowth, which locally penetrates the mucosal membrane, causing irritation and shedding of the tissues.

Yeasts that form buds are made of individual cells called blastospores or blastoconidia that reproduce by budding, although they occasionally reproduce through spore formation. A string of elongated buds called a pseudohypha can be formed that resembles a hyphal yeast form.

When *Candida* infects the mucous membranes of the oral cavity, it causes thrush. Thrush is characterized by a white speckling of the tongue and the back of the throat. Thrush is common in newborn babies, presumably caused by passage through an infected birth canal. It is also commonly seen in immunocompromised patients and individuals who have had a prolonged course of antibacterial therapy, reducing the normal bacterial population and allowing for the overgrowth of yeast.

Subcutaneous mycoses occur when *Candida* and other fungal species affect the dermis and underlying tissues. Systemic or generalized mycoses occur when fungal infections affect the internal organs of the body, occasionally affecting two or more different organ systems.

## Candida in Alzheimer's Disease

Amyloid beta protein has been found to have a particularly strong inhibitory activity against *C. albicans*. Thus, *C. albicans* infection causes a dramatic increase in amyloid beta protein. *C. albicans* is also known to cause protein misfolding, which can lead to the potent amyloid protein oligomers. In addition, several yeast and and other fungal proteins have been found to exhibit prion-like behavior in which the changes in phenotype were transmitted from mother to daughter cells in non-Mendelian fashion. This form of inheritance is driven by conversion of these proteins into amyloid fibrils and oligomers.

These findings led researchers to examine frozen brain specimens from AD patients to look for the presence of fungal elements. In their study, the researchers found fungal DNA and proteins in brain tissue from ten AD patients, but no fungal DNA or proteins were detected in ten control specimens (Pisa et al. 2015). The researchers then looked for the presence of fungi in tissue sections of the brain using frozen AD patient and control specimens. In particular, they examined the areas affected in AD, including the external frontal cortex, the cerebellar hemisphere, the entorhinal cortex/hippocampus and the choroid plexus. Using *C. glabrata* antibodies, they discovered fungal cells of variable size in neurons in these areas in samples from AD patients. No fungal cells were seen in the control samples. How-

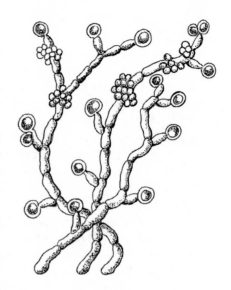

*Candida albicans.*

ever, the use of these antibodies doesn't indicate the fungi that the researchers found were from *C. glabrata* since other fungi are known to react with these antibodies (Pisa et al. 2015).

In another study designed to show the brain regions infected by fungi, researchers from Madrid studied the entorhinal cortex (the area of the brain that is first affected in AD) in samples from an AD patient, an elderly patient with no evidence of dementia, and one younger subject. In the patient with AD, a high number of various *C. albicans* structures were detected, whereas in the normal elderly subject, there were a small limited number of these structures. Conversely, the tissue from the young subject showed no evidence of fungal elements. Because the antibody used to detect the fungal elements can cross-react with other fungal species, other fungi besides *C. albicans* may have also been present (Alonso et al. 2018).

Additional testing of three AD patients and three control subjects in another study showed that several fungal species can infect blood vessels, resulting in vascular changes consistent with those seen in AD (Pisa et al. 2015).

Bodo Parady explains that the essence of AD development is the defeat of the innate immune system, whether through the patient's vulnerable health status or through treatment that suppresses inflammation, thereby also suppressing the innate immune system. With the discovery of the antimicrobial nature of amyloid beta protein, researchers can conjecture that the presence of amyloid may be evidence of the innate immune response that exists to destroy fungal colonization through structural interference and cytotoxicity (Parady 2018).

Parady explains the logic behind establishing a fungal contribution to AD. Because fungi can remain within cells for long periods, this situation can lead to a persistent state of reinfection. When the brain is injured, this persistent state is even more likely, and brain injury is known to result in AD. In addition, hyaline masses resulting from axonal injury known as corpora amylacea are known to develop independently in the brains of AD patients (Alonso et al. 2018). An analysis of the protein composition of corpora amylacea shows that the cells making up this structure were composed of fungal elements when the cells were still alive. These bodies require months or years to form, indicating that the fungal infection was present for a long time before the patient's death (Alonso et al. 2018).

Studies show the presence of *Alternia, Botyris, Candida, Cladosporium, Fusarium,* and *Malassezia* in AD-associated tissues. Of these, *Candida* is the most widespread, with *Candida* antibodies seen in 89.6 percent of AD patient serum compared to 8.8 percent in control subjects. Studies confirm that in mucosal *C. albicans* biofilms, a number of different bacteria coexist, including *Staphylococcus epidermis* (Adam et al. 2001). Biofilms are commonly seen in the amyloid beta plaques seen in AD. Biofilms are hardy and, when fungi are present, resistant to antibiotics.

AD and the motor neuron disease amyotrophic lateral sclerosis (ALS) share several clinical characteristics, including the accumulation of amyloid protein. In both AD and ALS, researchers have found evidence of fungal structures and DNA in cerebrospinal fluid samples. Further support for a disseminated fungal infection occurring in both AD and ALS comes from studies showing elevated levels of chitinase in the blood and cerebrospinal fluid in these patients before the manifestation of symptoms (Alonso et al. 2018).

## Molds

Molds are a type of fungus that can occasionally infect humans, especially patients with diabetes. Common bread molds that infect humans, such as *Rhizopus* and *Mucor,* are filamentous fungi belonging to the *Mucoraceae* family. These fungi have been known to infect immunosuppressed patients, causing the diseases zygomycosis in *Rhizopus* infection and mucormycosis in *Mucor* infection. Both *Mucor* and *Aspergillus* can grow in the walls of blood vessels, causing occlusion and tissue necrosis.

### *Cryptococcus neoformans* Infection

*Cryptococcus neoformans* (*C. neoformans*) is a fungus that causes dementia, and *C. neoformans* infection (Cryptococcosis) has been known to be occasionally misdiagnosed as Alzheimer's disease. Because *C. neoformans* exists as an encapsulated yeast, it has been confused with *Candida* infections. The India ink test traditionally used to diagnose *C. neoformans* is difficult to interpret and in recent years has largely been replaced by tests for the *C. neoformans* antigen.

*C. neoformans* is found in bird droppings, primarily from pigeons, chickens, and turkeys, as well as bat droppings. Because of its capsule, this fungus easily adheres to mucosal surfaces and is able to avoid phagocytosis by white blood cells. Infection usually presents as a subacute or chronic meningitis or as a pulmonary infection, which then spreads through the bloodstream to the brain. Infection of the lungs, kidneys, prostate, skin, and bone may also occur. Cryptococcosis is a common infection in Acquired Immune Deficiency Syndrome (AIDS) patients.

## Coexisting Bacterial Infections

Ruth Alonso, along with Luis Carrasco, has found a number of bacteria coexisting with fungi in the brains of AD patients. The most prevalent fungi in AD patients included *Alternaria, Botyris, Candida* and *Malassezia*. In control subjects, the most prominent fungi was *Fusarium*. In AD patients, the fungi present in the frontal cortex appear to be clustered together and differ markedly from any fungi present in control subjects (Alonso et al. 2018).

In both AD patients and controls, *Proteobacteria* was the most prominent bacteria, followed by *Firmicutes, Actinobacteria,* and *Bacteroidetes*. These happen to also be the four most prominent gut bacteria and collectively represent 98 percent of the gut bacteria. At the family level by classification, *Burkholderiaceae* and *Staphylococcaceae* were seen in higher percentages compared to control subjects.

## Protozoa

Protozoa are microorganisms belonging, along with algae, to the Kingdom *Protista*. Most protozoa are unicellular, although some are multicellular. Protozoa are classified by their mode of locomotion. Amoebas move by using their pseudopods (which, literally, mean "false feet"). Flagellates move by means of their whip-like flagella, and ciliates move by utilizing their hair-like cilia. Protozoa classified as *Sporozoa* do not have any motility extensions and exhibit no mobility.

Most protozoa, but not all, are parasites. Although most protozoal parasites of humans are obligate parasites, some species are facultive parasites, which means that they have the means to thrive on their own, but when they enter the human body, they become parasitic. The facultive amoeba *Acanthamoeba* species and *Naegleria fowleri*, for example, normally reside in soil or water, but when they enter the human body through the eyes or nasal mucosa, they travel via the olfactory nerve into the brain, causing diseases that affect the central nervous system (Engelkirk and Duben-Engelkirk 2015, 403).

# Toxoplasma gondii

*Toxoplasma gondii* (*T. gondii*) is an intracellular Sporozoan protozoa that causes the disease known as toxoplasmosis. The definitive hosts of *T. gondii* include cats that become infected after eating infected rodents or birds. Intermediate hosts include rodents, birds, sheep, goats, swine and cattle. Humans usually become infected when they eat infected raw or undercooked meat (usually pork or mutton) containing the cyst form of the parasite or by ingesting oocysts that have been shed in the feces of infected cats. Oocysts contain a zygote formed by a parasitic protozoa and indicate active protozoan replication.

*T. gondii* oocysts may be present in food or water contaminated by feline feces. Children have been known to accidentally ingest oocysts from sandboxes containing cat feces. Infection can also be acquired transplacentally from infected birth mothers, from blood transfusions, or through organ transplantation (Engelkirk and Duben-Engelkirk 2015, 405).

## *Toxoplasma gondii* in Alzheimer's Disease

Worldwide, one third of humans are infected with the brain-dwelling parasite *T. gondii*, with approximately fifteen million of these cases caused by congenital toxoplasmosis (Ngo et al. 2017). Neurobehavioral changes are seen in those who test positive for toxoplasmosis, although a direct cause for these changes has not yet been established. The susceptibility genes for congenital toxoplasmosis, however, are found in the human brain. Researchers, using systems biology approaches, have found associations between the interactions of the brain and *T. gondii* with epilepsy, movement disorders, Alzheimer's disease and cancer (Ngo et al. 2017).

The National Collaborative Chicago-based Congenital Toxoplasmosis Study (NCCCTS) has diagnosed, treated and followed 246 congenitally infected persons and their families continuously since 1981. Using data from NCCCTS, researchers have studied the genetic and parasitic effects that they hypothesized would affect patient outcomes (Ngo et al. 2017). To uncover potential developmental mechanisms related to neurodevelopment and neuroplasticity, they used neural stem cells infected with *T. gondii*. The researchers found that in the human host, dopamine and tyrosine hydroxylase were expressed in the neuronal cytoplasm. Alterations in their transmission led to the seizures that often occur in toxoplasmosis. As to why not all infected persons showed symptoms, the researchers hypothesized that the disease occurs when the relevant susceptibility genes are present, environmental factors (such as other infections) affect the immune system, and the parasites have a genotype conducive to aggressive infection (Ngo et al. 2017). Because all parasitic protozoa contain multiple protease enzymes, treatment that inhibits these enzymes is being studied as a potential treatment.

## Nematodes

Although they are not microorganisms, nematodes (also known as helminths) are parasitic worms that can enter the gastrointestinal system, circulatory system, central nervous system, eyes, muscles, and subcutaneous tissues. Similar to the entry of bacteria, viruses, fungi, and protozoa, helminths can enter the central nervous system through a defective blood-brain barrier.

The nematode *Caenorhabditis elegans* (*C. elegans*) has been widely used as an animal model of Alzheimer's disease. Researchers often first try out promising drugs on *C. elegans* worms before introducing them to human subjects.

However, worms have also been found in the central nervous system, gastrointestinal tract, vascular system, eyes and skin, where they cause a number of diseases, including dementia. For instance, cysts from the larval stage of the pork tapeworm (*Taenia solium*) have been found in the brain, causing the helminth disease cysticercosis. Hydatid cysts from *Echinococcus granulosis* and *Echinococcus multilocularis* are found in the brain and other locations in the body (Engelkirk and Duben-Engelkirk 2015, 413).

The first description of a parasitic infestation in AD has been found in the postmortem brain specimens from five patients with AD. The tissue specimens were obtained from the Harvard University Brain Tissue Resource Center and contained neural *Larva migrans* worms containing *Borrelia* microbes. Because these helminths and associated spirochetes were first seen in Lewy body dementia, researchers went on to study the brains of AD patients. *Larva migrans* usually attacks the skin, resulting in a condition of cutaneous larva migrans, which is caused by the larvae of various nematode parasites of the hookworm family (*Ancylostomatidae*). While more studies are needed, these parasites are known to cause the neuroinflammation characteristic of AD (MacDonald 2016).

## Summary

A large number of fungi, molds, parasitic protozoa, and helminths have been found in the brains of AD subjects. Often accompanied by bacteria, viruses, or bacteriophages in the biofilms that cover plaques, these organisms are thought to contribute to the neuroinflammation, neurodegeneration, and increased abundance of amyloid beta plaque seen in AD.

# TEN

# Risk Factors

A number of lifestyle, dietary, metabolic, and infectious causes have been found to be associated with the development of Alzheimer's disease and are considered risk factors. However, not everyone with risk factors goes on to develop AD. Defying the odds, some individuals with AD appear to have lived lives that suggested they would be totally free from cognitive decline. However, in most cases, following a healthy lifestyle and avoiding known risk factors helps in preserving cognitive function. Although two copies of the APOE-ε4 allele are reported to cause a nine-fold increase in AD in people of European descent, the vast majority of people with the APOE-ε4 allele don't develop AD, and about half of AD patients do not have an APOE-ε4 allele (Rose and Rose 2012, 88). Consequently, risk factors play a larger-than-expected role.

As the Cornell immunotoxicologist Rodney Dietert explains, the introduction of antibiotics and vaccines greatly reduced the risk of developing infectious diseases. However, their use has led to an increase in non-communicable diseases, including all cancers, thyroid disorders, allergies, depression, and Alzheimer's disease. These diseases kill three times as many people as the infectious diseases would have (Dietert 2016, 7). The two fallacies that led to this increase are the notion that we're better off without microbes and the notion that our genes are the most important biologic factor governing our health. The consequences of this situation are described later in this chapter.

## Studying Risk Factors

Today it's known that women are twice as likely as men to develop Alzheimer's disease. Latinos are 1.5 more likely to have Alzheimer's disease than Caucasians, and African Americans are 2–3 times more likely to develop Alzheimer's disease than other populations. In addition, veterans who have suffered traumatic brain injuries are 60 percent more likely to develop Alzheimer's disease (Vradenburg 2019).

Studying the habits of populations with a low incidence of Alzheimer's disease is a first-line approach to identifying risk factors. Chapman University has recently been awarded an additional $2.9 million, raising its total grants from the National Institutes of Health/National Institute on Aging to $6.9 million (Chapman University 2018). These research grants are for the Tsimane Health and Life History Project, a study of brain aging in the Tsimane people in Bolivia (Gurven et al. 2017). The Tsimane have a low incidence of both cardiovascular disease and Alzheimer's disease and at one time were said to have the lowest incidence of AD in the world.

In the second part of their study, the researchers will evaluate the neighboring Moseten tribe, a similar population characterized by individuals with a low incidence of cardiovascular disease, although they exhibit more variation in lifestyle and metabolic risk factors. (See more on the Tsimane people in the "Infection and Microglial Activation" section of this chapter.)

In 2002, the average life expectancy for the Tsimane had increased to 53 years. With aging as the most important risk factor for late-onset Alzheimer's disease (LOAD), it is difficult to compare their low incidence of AD to that of individuals in industrialized countries. However, we can learn a great deal from studying the immune system's response to infection in the Tsimane population compared to the immune response in infection typically seen in the United States and Europe, which have the highest incidences of AD in the world.

## Aging

Aging is the greatest risk factor for developing AD. After age 65, the likelihood of developing Alzheimer's doubles about every five years, and after age 85, the risk reaches nearly 50 percent. Aging itself is associated with several physiological changes that increase AD risk. With inflammaging, the immune system is no longer as robust. One of the hallmarks of aging is the shortening of the telomeres found at the ends of chromosomes. Human CD4 T lymphocytes lose about 3,000 bp of their telomeric sequences between ages 20 and 60. Then the length of telomeres plateaus out to a total length of 5,000–6,000. These older T cells, aware of their precarious situation, are no longer capable of participating in a robust immune response (Weyand and Goronzy 2016). Short telomeres, which can result from radiation-induced genetic mutations and occur as a result of aging, are associated with a shorter lifespan. Ways to increase telomere length are described in Chapter Twelve.

With aging, the risk of infection is more common and becomes more difficult to treat. In addition, the blood-brain barrier and the gut's intestinal barrier both become more permeable, which gives microbes greater opportunity to make their way into the central nervous system. Medications commonly used for pain and arthritis in the elderly can also injure the intestinal and brain barriers and cause an ineffective immune response. While aging certainly can't be prevented, there are many factors that influence how well people age.

An individual's general health is a good measure of brain health. When blood pressure, cholesterol, and glucose levels are under control, the vascular system remains healthy and the immune system is efficient. While genetics have some impact on general health, most of the risk factors associated with aging are considered modifiable.

## Diet and Nutrition

Excess sugar consumption has been found to have the most significant effect on the development and progression of Alzheimer's disease. Besides its lack of nutrients, the metabolism of sugar depletes magnesium, B vitamins and many other nutrients. Since 1900, the average ingestion of sugar has grown from five pounds annually (mostly from fruit) to 190 pounds annually (primarily from refined sugar) (Sherzai and Sherzai 2017, 101). Excess sugar is directly responsible for elevated triglycerides, hypertension, blood vessel inflammation, insulin resistance, metabolic syndrome, and diabetes—all conditions that increase the risk for AD.

A Mediterranean diet is widely recommended for the prevention of AD and for good general health. The Mediterranean diet is rich in fruits, vegetables, olive oil, legumes, whole grains (if tolerated), nuts, and fish— foods rich in nutrients and low in sugar and saturated fats. In a Columbia University study, the risk of dying from AD was 73 percent lower in individuals who strictly adhered to the Mediterranean diet and 35 percent lower in those who only followed the diet moderately (Sherzai and Sherzai 2017, 93).

When following any diet, it's important to avoid eating known and suspected allergens and foods that are genetically modified, processed, or contaminated with glyphosate and other pesticides. While organic fruits and vegetables are generally considered superior, rinsing produce well is also important. Many people have trouble digesting today's grains, which bear little resemblance to the grains adopted by ancient hunter-gatherer societies. Besides gluten and lectins in seeds, today's grains are likely to contain azodicarbonamide, glyphosate and other chemicals that disrupt our immune system. It's no wonder that leading researchers recommend avoiding grains (Perlmutter 2013, 63–65; Bredesen 2017, 46–48; Gundry 2019, 32).

The Chicago Health and Aging Project, a longitudinal study of the factors that contribute to chronic disease involving 2,500 older subjects, found that those individuals who consumed higher amounts of saturated and trans fatty acids over a 6-year period had a higher risk for AD compared to individuals who favored plant-based fat sources (Sherzai and Sherzai 2017, 86).

Harvard researchers for the Women's Health Study also found that a higher saturated fat intake was associated with a faster decline in memory. Women with the greatest intake of saturated fats, particularly from red meats, had nearly a 70 percent higher risk of cognitive impairment. Women with the lowest intake of saturated fats had the brain function of women who were six years younger (Sherzai and Sherzai 2017, 87).

Low levels of vitamin B12, vitamin B1, vitamin B6, folate, vitamin D, vitamin A, and vitamin E can all cause conditions of dementia and lead to a diagnosis of Alzheimer's disease.

Certain medications, including proton pump inhibitors and non-steroidal anti-inflammatory drugs, cause an increased risk for AD by disrupting the epithelial lining of the gut, resulting in leaky gut syndrome, which can contribute to nutrient deficiencies. Microbes are also known to ingest various medications, which can reduce nutrients administered as dietary supplements.

## Family History

Among people with early-onset familial AD (EOFAD) who have one of the three rare mutations associated with EOFAD (described later in this chapter), patients have 50 percent chance of inheriting the mutation. Among those with late-onset AD (LOAD), individuals who have the APOE-ε4 gene and who also have one parent or two siblings with AD have an increased risk of developing LOAD.

Genetic counselors often ask patients about grandparents, aunts, uncles, and great aunts and uncles to help prepare a more detailed view of genetic risk.

## Stress and Lifestyle

One's lifestyle, including reactions to stress, as well as one's social connections, education, habits, hobbies and sleep patterns, also influence cognitive health. Stress is neither inherently good nor bad, although any stressor (even the stress of winning the lottery) can be overwhelming. Resilient individuals react to acute and chronic stress, including a serious accident or injury or a long-term goal, by responding appropriately and moving on. In lingering over acute stressors or dealing inappropriately with chronic stress, the immune system becomes weakened and no longer launches an appropriate response. Studies have demonstrated that the effects of lingering or chronic stress can injure brain structures as well. Stress reduction techniques, including biofeedback, meditation, tai chi, and exercise, can reduce the effects of stress and serve as beneficial coping strategies. Uncontrolled stress can inhibit the production of serotonin and lead to anxiety and depression, both of which are risk factors for AD (Sherzai and Sherzai 2017, 182).

The gut microbiome also affects an individual's response to stress and social anxiety, primarily through its production of neurotransmitters and neuromodulators, particularly serotonin and gamma-aminobutyric acid. The gut microbiome and the chemicals it produces also directly affect the physiology of the brain (Dietert 2016, 243).

## Social Connections

Numerous studies have emphasized the importance of social connections for mental health. Having a sense of community, keeping up with family ties, belonging to productive online or local social groups, and meeting up with old friends can all benefit cognitive health.

Studies of the Tsimane tribe, which is a contemporary, isolated, nonindustrial population, show how changes that add complexity (such as having a cash economy) can also alter health. Although there are 36 indigenous groups that constitute 60 percent of the population in Colombia, the Tsimane are the most isolated. The members are forager-horticulturists who grow a variety of plants such as plantains and rice; fish in the nearby streams, rivers and lagoons; and gather fruits and other foods such as nuts and honey. The Tsimane population is exceptional because of its low incidence of cardiovascular disease and Alzheimer's disease. Their activity level is high, and they live in a close social community.

In their work as co-directors of the Brain Health and Alzheimer's Prevention Program at Loma Linda University, Dean and Ayesha Sherzai explain that social behaviors, especially complex interactions, work on many levels to increase cognitive reserve. For instance, complex communication skills involve different brain functions, including face recognition, memory, focus, attention, and both auditory and language skills. Social interactions also generate emotions that are important for motivation and for finding meaning in life. They have likewise found that social interaction decreases depression and low mood states, and it encourages people to engage in activities (such as exercise) that they might hesitate to do alone (Sherzai and Sherzai 2017, 256).

## Education and Hobbies

Numerous studies show that formal education in early life correlates with a higher cognitive reserve in the elderly population. Even educational advances achieved in people older than 60 years have been shown to improve cognitive performance. Complexity is important, and people with hobbies that require learning can offset the neurological damage caused by a poor diet (Sherzai and Sherzai 2017, 261). Studies show that dance classes, exercise routines, learning a musical instrument, learning new languages, journal writ-

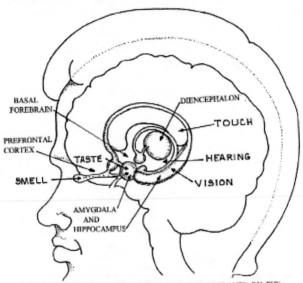

STIMULUS RECEIVED BY THE CEREBRAL CORTEX IS RELAYED BY THE AMYGDALA AND HIPPOCAMPUS TO THE DIENCEPHALON. THE INFORMATION IS NEXT TRANSMITTED TO THE PREFRONTAL CORTEX AND THE BASAL FOREBRAIN. WHERE IT IS TRANSMITTED BACK TO THE SAME SENSORY AREA THAT FIRST RECEIVED THE INFORMATION. SOME MEMORY MAY BE STORED IN THE CEREBRAL CORTEX DURING THIS PROCESS.

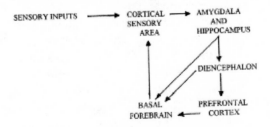

**Learning Thought Process.**

ing, participating in singing groups, mentoring others, volunteering in one's community or online, and becoming involved in the care of grandchildren or other young family members can also improve cognitive reserve.

Hobbies give individuals a sense of purpose as they work to complete projects. Hobbies also provide opportunities for meeting new people and participating in both local and online communities.

## Sleep

Sleep deprivation is a risk factor for Alzheimer's disease. During sleep, amyloid beta protein is cleared from the brain. In experimental models of AD, sleep deprivation has been found to increase the concentration of soluble amyloid beta (Aβ) protein, resulting in a chronic accumulation of Aβ protein in the brain, whereas subjects who typically sleep 7–8 hours each night do not show these accumulations. Sleep disorders are a common feature in patients with AD and are seen in the early course of the disease. Rapid eye movement appears to decrease as the disease progresses.

In addition, research suggests that averaging less than six hours of sleep per night is associated with the development of amyloid plaques as well as increases in brain levels of tau protein in cognitively normal individuals (McKeehan 2019). In one study, participants with the highest levels of tau protein (measured by brain imaging or spinal fluid levels) had the lowest levels of non-rapid eye movement sleep, which is the part of sleep important for forming long-term memories (McKeehan 2019). Because changes in amyloid and tau proteins develop at least a decade before symptoms of cognitive impairment occur, these changes may be early manifestations of AD.

## Hearing Loss

Researchers at Johns Hopkins University report that individuals with hearing loss are 24 percent more likely to develop Alzheimer's disease. In studies, researchers found that the more severe the hearing loss, the more likely the person was to develop dementia. The reasons for this result are unclear, although researchers suspect that hearing loss itself can lead to social isolation (Hicks 2018). More studies are needed to see whether hearing loss is related to ear infections that patients experienced as children. Hearing loss caused by changes associated with infection is known as conductive hearing loss.

## Head Injuries

Although the majority of head injuries are mild, the most common is a non-repetitive traumatic brain injury (TBI). An analysis of seven studies of patients followed for one year after sustaining a TBI found that although TBI was not associated with increased risk of all types of dementia, there was an increased risk of AD (Livingston et al. 2017). In addition, repetitive mild head injury among athletes or soldiers is associated with a condition of chronic traumatic encephalopathy, which is a progressive condition of increased cerebral tau protein that can eventually progress to dementia. The Institute of Medicine (IOM) has concluded that moderate or severe TBI is a risk factor for AD.

A study by the IOM found that TBI-induced neurovascular injuries accelerate Aβ production and deposits, arterial stiffness, tau hyperphosphorylation, and tau/Aβ-induced blood-brain barrier damage, which are predisposing factors for AD (Ramos-Cejudo et al. 2018).

## Gut Dysbiosis

Alterations in the gut microbiome are commonly seen in patients with AD, and these alterations lead to defects in the gut's protective lining. In Alzheimer's disease, phylogenetic diversity in the gut microbiome is decreased, which leads to an imbalance of neurotransmitters, hormones, vitamins, and other chemicals produced by gut microbes. At the phylum level, individuals with AD had decreases in the presence of *Firmicutes* as a whole, with decreases seen in several microbial families and genera. These decreases are also seen in individuals with obesity and type 2 diabetes, which are both risk factors for AD (Vogt et al. 2017). The gut microbiota in AD is likewise characterized by a decreased abundance of *Bifidobacterium* and an increased abundance of *Bacteroidetes*.

Leaky gut syndrome caused by alterations in the gut microbiota allows for the passage of microbes and lipopolysaccharides into the central nervous system. However, a corrective program of rebiosis based on dietary changes, prebiotics and probiotics can restore the health of the gut microbiome. The gut microbiota plays an important role in the production of signaling molecules, hormones, and neurotransmitters. Disruptions in the gut microbiome that disrupt as little as 1 percent of the microbial population can result in anxiety, autoimmune diseases, metabolic syndrome, obesity and stress-induced and progressive neuropsychiatric diseases such as schizophrenia and Alzheimer's disease (Hill et al. 2014). Several studies show improvement in cognitive function following the use of probiotics.

### Immune System Effects

Hippocrates once said that all diseases originate in the gut. While this may not always be the case, the gut plays a vital role in the maintenance of health. Metabolites produced by gut microbes have been found to modulate the immune system. The intestinal (enteric) immune system is known to have co-evolved with the gut microbiota for the maintenance of intestinal health. Intestinal microbes are essential for digestion as well as the production of numerous chemicals and metabolites. For this reason, the gut is often referred to as an endocrine organ, the second brain, or the second liver.

In one example of the effects of microbes on the enteric immune system, researchers have found that *Bacteroides fragilis* and *Clostridium* species lead to regulatory T cells (Tregs) in the colon. The short-chain fatty acids and gut-derived fermentation products of these bacteria regulate the number and function of these cells. In doing so, Tregs that express the transcription factor Foxp3 offer protection against colitis (Smith et al. 2013).

## Glyphosate and GMO Foods

Glyphosate is an organophosphorus compound with antibiotic properties first introduced in 1974 and widely used as an herbicide. Products containing glyphosate usually contain other substances that can strengthen the potency of organophosphorus compounds. Glyphosate is also part of the strategy in producing genetically modified organisms (GMOs), which are designed to produce glyphosate-resistant crops (Dietert 2016, 256).

Recent studies show that glyphosate reduces the presence of soil fungi that are symbiotic with grass roots needed to support foraging animals. Glyphosate can also alter the susceptibility or resistance to antibiotics in pathogenic bacteria. In a study of chickens, pathogenic bacteria were more resistant to glyphosate than any of the helpful commensal bacteria. An increase in botulism-related disease in cattle seen in recent years is related to glyphosate's suppression of the antagonistic effect of *Enterococcus* species on *Clostridium botulinum* (Dietert 2016, 256).

In a 2018 study conducted by researchers at Indiana University and the University of California, San Francisco, 71 pregnant women were tested for the presence of glyphosate in their urine. Detectable levels of glyphosate were found in 93 percent of the urine samples (Gundry 2019, 31–32).

The problems caused by glyphosate are numerous, and more studies are showing its adverse effects. Glyphosate destroys the gut microbiome and disrupts the tight intestinal barrier, leading to leaky gut syndrome. As an antibiotic, glyphosate kills bacteria and disrupts the ability of gut microbes to produce the essential acids tryptophan and phenylalanine (needed to produce serotonin), as well as thyroid hormone (Gundry 2019, 31). Glyphosate is found in fresh produce and in the meat and milk of animals that are fed grains and beans.

## *Infection and Microglial Activation*

In recent years, the Tsimane people have been recognized as having a very low incidence of Alzheimer's disease, a situation that may be related to their lifestyle, which includes being physically active for eight hours or longer each day. (A lack of exercise is a known risk factor for AD.) The Tsimane also live a relatively isolated existence. They only marry within the tribe and have few modern conveniences. In addition, they have a low prevalence of diabetes, hypertension and cardiovascular disease, although they are burdened by infectious and inflammatory conditions and have a high infant mortality rate.

At least 66 percent of the Tsimane people are infected with parasites at any given time, and anthropologists think this was most likely true for our ancestors as well (Gurven et al. 2017). The prevalence of parasites is also high in India, a country with a low incidence of Alzheimer's disease. Researchers are studying whether the infections caused by the parasites could change the way genes act in our bodies, or if APOE-ε4 actually played a survival role in ancient times, defending the brain from pathogenic parasites and infections.

Researchers have also found that the Tsimane members with infections were more likely to maintain cognitive fitness if they carried at least one copy of the APOE-ε4 gene. The individuals free of parasitic infection who had the APOE-ε4 gene experienced cognitive decline, just like people in industrialized countries today (Gurven et al. 2017).

Even those Tsimane members who have one or two APOE-ε4 alleles do not appear to be affected by Alzheimer's disease and appear to perform better than others in their group on cognitive tests. Researchers are currently focusing on the role of inflammation as a contributor to Alzheimer's disease. However, as seen in other societies, the influx of Western civilization is causing changes that may bear on this study. Cell phones and canned foods have recently been introduced to the Tsimane population. But much can still be learned, particularly whether the APOE-ε4 gene (like the sickle cell mutation that offers protection against malaria) prevents parasites and microbes from entering the central nervous system.

### Microglial Activation

A number of infectious agents described in this book are associated with the development of AD. Numerous researchers have described the first case of AD noted by Alois Alzheimer as a condition of meningoencephalitis caused by *Mycobacterium tuberculosis*. Activated microglial cells related to infection, which are a characteristic feature in AD, are known to damage neurons and cause the changes seen in Alzheimer's patient Auguste Deter (Broxmeyer 2016, 14).

Animal models show that when activated microglia are further activated by a subsequent systemic infection, levels of interleukin-1 beta increase and lead to neurodegeneration. In animal models of Alzheimer's disease, researchers found that cognitive function can be impaired for at least two months after the successful treatment of a systemic infection (Holmes et al. 2003).

In AD patients who develop a systemic infection, delirium is often seen, which further impairs their cognitive state. In older patients, delirium is an independent predictor of sustained poor cognition after one year, and of dementing illness when it persists for two years or longer. This systemic response is also characterized by a rise in the cytokines interleukin-6 and interleukin-1 beta. In a study of 85 patients with AD, researchers predicted that, as in the animal models, systemic infection would lead to persistent cognitive decline accompanied by microglial activation and a rise in pro-inflammatory cytokines. The results of their study indicated that both systemic infection and increased levels of interleukin-1 beta in serum caused by microglial activation are associated with a greater rate of cognitive decline (Holmes et al. 2003).

## Environmental Toxins

From 1935 through 1985, Dupont's advertising slogan "Better Living Through Chemistry" dominated the headlines. Dichlorodiphenyltrichloroethane (DDT) was the first of the pesticides, and it was used liberally by soldiers in World War II as a preventive measure against malaria and typhus. Although it was known that DDT crippled the nervous systems of insects, it was decades later when scientists learned that DDT disrupts the endocrine system of humans. To compound the problem, by 1952, nearly 10,000 new pesticides had been introduced in the United States. The effects of pesticides have been mixed, with most studies showing decreased biodiversity, harmful algal blooms caused by toxicity to certain algae and diatoms, and alterations in ecosystem food webs.

As for the effects on cognitive function, strong evidence shows that industrial chemicals that have been widely disseminated in the environment have contributed to the pandemic of neurodevelopmental toxicity. In adults, most neurological deficits are caused by an acute exposure seen in workers (as described in the next section), while during development these chemicals can cause permanent brain injury with low levels of exposure. Expectant mothers exposed to chlorpyrifos (which continues to be sprayed on apples in the United States) were found to have children with smaller head circumferences at birth—an indication of slowed brain growth in utero—and with neurobehavioral deficits that persisted for up to seven years (Grandjean and Landrigan 2014).

Organochlorine compounds such as DDT and chlordecone are highly persistent and remain widespread in the environment and in the bodies of humans. The cord blood of newborns has been reported to contain an average of 280 chemicals, including organochlorine compounds. The major problem is that most chemicals are assumed to be safe despite having never been tested for safety. Phillipe Grandjean and Philip Landrigan describe the classic examples of chemicals that were never tested for safety and later found to have major adverse effects, including asbestos, thalidomide, diethylstilbestrol, and chlorofluorocarbons.

The effects of pesticides are difficult to predict. Some species have been found to be adversely affected, whereas others are able to break down pesticides and use the chemical components as nutrients. Either way, pesticides can alter the human microbiome.

## Aluminum

For the past 40 years, aluminum has been implicated in the development of AD, but there are too many conflicting studies to state that aluminum is a cause of AD. However, studies of individuals who died from familial AD show high brain concentrations of aluminum. More likely, aluminum has an effect similar to that of mercury and can cause dementia when individuals are exposed to large amounts.

In February 2014, researchers at Keele University in the United Kingdom reported the first case of an individual who was occupationally exposed to aluminum and died from early-onset AD. The patient was a 58-year-old man who worked for eight years in the preparation of an insulating material for nuclear fuel. His occupation exposed him to aluminum sulphate particles. Within a short time of starting this work, the patient complained of headaches, fatigue and mouth ulcers. He died at age 66, and a postmortem examination confirmed Alzheimer's disease. The aluminum content of his frontal lobe was assessed in 49 different tissue samples. The aluminum levels were four times higher than that seen in age-matched controls (Keele University 2014).

Although abundant in the environment, aluminum is not essential for life and is considered a neurotoxin known to inhibit more than 200 important biological functions. It was first reported to be associated with memory disorders in 1921. In recent years, aluminum exposure has been found to cause dialysis encephalopathy and is suspected of contributing to amyotrophic lateral sclerosis, Parkinson's dementia in the Kii Peninsula, Gulf War syndrome, and AD (Kawahara and Kato-Negishi 2011).

Researchers have found that aluminum, iron, zinc, and copper may all contribute to the production of the toxic amyloid beta oligomers seen in AD. Aluminum in particular binds to a number of metal-binding proteins and can result in these conformational changes. Aluminum is known to have adverse effects on the mammalian nervous system, including developmental defects in axon transport, neurotransmitter synthesis, gene expression and inflammatory responses.

The accidental contamination of aluminum in drinking water exposed 20,000 individuals to high levels of aluminum in 1988 in the United Kingdom. In a 10-year follow-up study, those affected exhibited various symptoms of cerebral impairment, including a loss of concentration and defects in short-term memory. In addition, areas with high concentrations of aluminum in drinking water in England and Wales reported a high incidence of AD. Similar cases were reported in Norway and Canada (Kawahara and Kato-Negishi 2011). High concentrations of aluminum are also associated with high-fat/high-energy diets (Goschorska et al. 2018).

Matrix metalloproteinases are enzymes that facilitate the binding of metals such as aluminum and copper to proteins, including amyloid beta protein. High levels of matrix metalloproteinases are known to increase the risk of developing AD. Therapies to reduce the level of these enzymes are under development (Stromrud et al. 2010).

As for its effects on microbes and the gut microbiome, in the oligodynamic effect, some metals (such as silver) are known to kill off microbes and are especially well suited for cooking utensils. Aluminum is known to cause bacteria to flourish (Fenlon 2013).

## Mercury

Acute mercury exposure or chronic exposure to low levels of inorganic mercury has long been known to cause dementia. Several studies show elevated concentrations of mercury in the brains of AD patients that are suspected of being related to dental amalgams. Patients with dental amalgams contain 2–10 times the amount of mercury seen in the brains of AD patients without fillings. Dental amalgam consists of 50 percent elementary mercury, which is constantly being vaporized and absorbed (Mutter et al. 2010).

The high affinity of mercury for selenium suggests that mercury may lead to neurodegenerative disorders by disrupting redox regulation, which leads to an increased production of reactive oxygen species, a known cause of neuroinflammation and neurodegeneration. If high levels of organic and inorganic mercury are seen, chelation can effectively remove them, particularly the Quicksilver method, which uses pulsed treatments. Amalgam fillings should be removed by a biological dentist to avoid exposing patients to high levels of mercury generated during the removal process.

# Fluoride

Since the 1940s, fluoride has been added to numerous drinking water supplies in an effort to decrease the rate of tooth decay. In recent years, it's been found that improved hygiene may the reason for the improvement in dental health rather than fluoride, which is a known neurotoxin. Excess fluoride is known to cause accumulations of fluoride in bone, causing brittle bones; dental fluorosis, which causes tooth discoloration and pitting; and hypothyroidism as iodine is displaced by fluoride. Fluoride is also known to affect the developing brain, and high fluoride levels are associated with reduced IQ scores.

Fluoride is able to cross the blood-brain barrier, especially when it binds with aluminum molecules. In the brain, fluoride affects cellular energy metabolism, the synthesis of pro-inflammatory factors, microglial activation, and neurotransmitter metabolism (Goschorska et al. 2018). Fluoride also tends to accumulate in the hippocampus, where it impairs memory formation.

Fluoride has been linked to many steps in the process of neuroinflammation, most notably stimulation of cytokine secretion and activation of macrophages and microglia. Fluoride is also known to increase acute-phase reactant proteins. In addition, fluoride results in stimulation of the pro-inflammatory cytokines IL-1 beta, IL-2, IL-6, and TNF-alpha. Fluoride likewise stimulates the activity of phospholipase A2 and cyclooxygenases, features seen in AD.

Declan Waugh describes the lower brain levels of acetylcholinesterase activity that are seen in the cognitive impairment of adults. Because fluoride is known to reduce levels of this enzyme, the lowering of acetylcholinesterase is another link to AD. In 2014, the National Academy of Sciences in India reported that exposure to fluoride results in significant impairment of acetylcholinesterase activity, with the maximum inhibition occurring in the brain. The study also found that co-exposure to fluoride and the chlorpyrifos pesticide that is still used in the United States resulted in synergistic toxicity or enhanced impairment of acetylcholinesterase activity (Waugh 2018).

Waugh also describes a 2015 study that found that drinking water containing recommended levels of fluoride resulted in brain neurotoxicity by causing severe neuronal changes and impairing acetylcholinesterase activity in the brain.

# Ionizing Radiation

Considerable evidence shows that amyloid beta protein accumulations in AD result from increased production or reduced clearance. These protein aggregates are associated with inflammation, oxidative stress and neuronal loss. More than twenty years ago, researchers proposed that reactive oxygen species were the main cause of AD because neurons in AD patients exhibit signs of chronic oxidative stress, including oxidative RNA damage. The association of APOE and several new genes (such as CD33m, CLU, and BIN1) in late-onset AD also suggests that the immune response and sterol and lipid metabolism could be involved.

Because ionizing radiation (IR) has been found to cause physiological and cognitive effects when high doses are used, a team of researchers from Bangladesh and Japan conducted an animal study using mice to see the effects of lower doses of IR and determine how these might apply to the development of AD (Begum et al. 2012).

Actively dividing cells are known to be more sensitive to IR, and children exposed to prenatal radiation show evidence of learning disabilities and mental retardation. IR is also known to lead to vascular abnormalities, demyelination, disruptions of the blood-brain barrier and alterations in the brain's microenvironment.

The researchers concluded that because IR accelerates aging (a risk factor for AD), there is consistent evidence that IR might trigger mechanisms that lead to AD development (Begum et al. 2012).

## Homocysteine Levels

Vascular defects, including hypertension and atrial fibrillation, are known to increase the incidence of vascular dementia as well as AD. Elevated homocysteine levels, which frequently occur in methylenetetrahydrofolate reductase (MTHFR) mutations, are associated with an increased risk of atherosclerosis, death from cardiovascular causes, coronary heart disease, carotid atherosclerosis and stroke. Because of these findings, researchers conducted a study and discovered that elevated plasma homocysteine levels are associated with an increased risk of AD.

The subjects were also tested for vitamin B6, vitamin B12, and folate (folic acid) levels. Deficiencies in all three of these B vitamins have previously been associated with elevated homocysteine levels. However, after adjusting for these levels, none were independently related to the risk of vascular dementia or AD. The researchers found that an increment in the plasma homocysteine level of 5 umol/L increased the risk of AD by 40 percent. A plasma homocysteine level in the highest age-specific quartile doubled the risk of AD (Seshadri et al. 2002; Goschorska et al. 2018).

## The APOE-ε4 Gene and Lipids

Lipid disturbances are an important risk factor for AD. The ε4 allele of the apolipoprotein E (APOE) gene, which is the strongest genetic risk factor for sporadic AD, is highly associated with lipid metabolism. The APOE gene instructs the body to produce apolipoprotein E, which combines with lipids present in the body to form molecules known as lipoproteins. Lipoproteins package cholesterol and other fatty substances and carry them through the bloodstream. APOE is known to encode a specific protein that regulates cholesterol metabolism in the brain as well as the body's metabolism of triglyceride. Within the brain, cholesterol is primarily found in its unesterified form in myelin sheaths and in the cellular membranes of neurons and glial cells.

The lipid profile seen in the majority of patients with AD includes a total cholesterol higher than 200 mg/dL, an elevated low-density lipoprotein (LDL) level, and an elevated triglyceride level with a normal high-density lipoprotein (HDL) level and total cholesterol/HDL ratio. While statin cholesterol-lowering medications have been shown to reduce amyloid beta protein levels, they have not resulted in cognitive improvement. The pathways of lipid metabolism appear to have a greater involvement.

Dysregulation of lipid pathways is a feature of many neurodegenerative disorders, including AD. This dysregulation has a direct effect on synaptic signaling, the processing of amyloid precursor protein, and the production of neurofibrillary tangles.

The gut microbiota has been found to have an effect on cardiovascular disease. Dysbiosis in the gut increases the permeability of the gut lining. This condition leads to increased blood levels of bacterial products, including lipopolysaccharides, which cause low-grade chronic inflammation (hypothesized to lead to insulin resistance and associated effects on lipid levels) (Fu et al. 2015).

In a study of the relationship of gut microbes to lipids, researchers found that the gut microbiome influences body mass index (BMI), triglyceride levels, and high-density lipoproteins (Fu et al. 2015). Previous studies have shown improvement in metabolic syndrome after altering the gut microbiome. Specific associations with microbes include the fact that a lower BMI is associated with a higher abundance of *Akkermansia*, which is increased by the drug metformin; a higher abundance of the genus *Eggerthella* is associated with increased triglyceride and decreased HDL levels; and an abundance of the genus *Butyricimonas* is associated with lower triglyceride levels (Fu et al. 2015). Probiotics and dietary changes can alter the gut microbiome.

## Summary

Various risk factors have been associated with the development of AD, with aging at the top of the list. Overall, most of the risk factors for AD

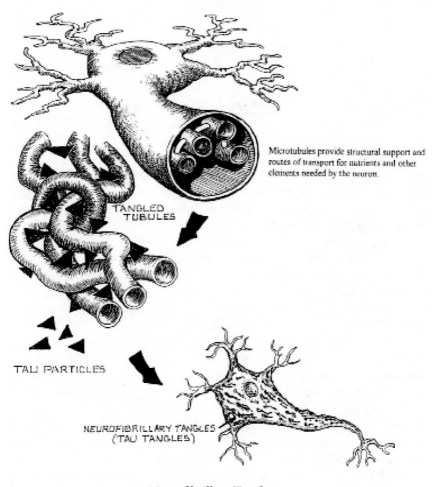

Microtubules provide structural support and routes of transport for nutrients and other elements needed by the neuron.

TANGLED TUBULES

TAU PARTICLES

NEUROFIBRILLARY TANGLES (TAU TANGLES)

**Neurofibrillary Tangles.**

are modifiable through alterations in the gut microbiome, diet, exercise, lifestyle and the addition of dietary supplements, particularly antioxidants. This chapter describes the many risk factors that are associated with AD and the ways in which these factors contribute to the physiological changes that occur in AD.

# ELEVEN

# Genetic Influences

When the Human Genome Project was first proposed, it was widely predicted that humans would have more genes than smaller organisms and that most diseases would be highly associated with genes. This has not been the case. Sequencing the three billion nucleotides of the human genome, a process completed in 2003, was certainly a triumph of technological ingenuity. However, it ultimately led to the discovery that the cells' internal regulatory processes control what genes are activated at the critical times needed for human development. Consequently, it became clear that cells play a more important role in terms of human development than genes (Rose and Rose 2012, 72).

Despite the lofty expectations of the scientists involved in the project, humans have been found to have approximately 22,000 genes, compared to 20,000 in roundworms and 31,000 in tiny water fleas. When DNA insertions and deletions are taken into account, human still share 96 percent of their DNA sequence with chimpanzees.

It's also now known that single genes have minimal influence, and only about 2 percent of genetic diseases are directly caused by a single gene (Heine 2017, 36). In addition, genes only have a 20–30 percent impact on the development of most diseases, with diet, lifestyle and other environmental factors playing a much greater role. The strongest single genetic predictor of a common disease is the relation between the APOE gene and Alzheimer's disease risk (Heine 2017, 87).

In Alzheimer's disease, genes play a limited role. There is no one gene specifically associated with AD development. In early-onset AD (EOAD), which occurs before age 65 and represents less than 5 percent of all cases of AD, several genes are associated with disease development and thus have greater influence than the genes associated with sporadic or late-onset AD (LOAD). In LOAD, the role of genes is more tenuous, and the APOE-ε4 gene, which has the most significant association with AD, has its own association with microbes.

**170**

## Genes and Gene Mutations

Francis Crick and Jim Watson became famous when they discovered deoxyribonucleic acid (DNA) in 1953. DNA is composed of the four small molecules or nucleotides—adenine, cytosine, guanine, and thymine—connected to a sugar (deoxyribose) and a phosphate molecule. The sequence of these nucleotides makes up the individual's genetic code. In humans, the DNA that constitutes genes is located within 23 pairs of chromosomes, one strand handed down from the mother and one strand from the father. These chromosomes are present in the DNA found within the nucleus of nearly every cell within the body. In addition to this nuclear DNA, cell

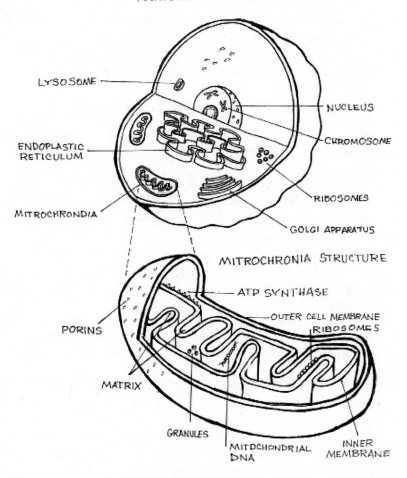

**Cell and Mitochondria.**

mitochondria contain mitochondrial DNA, which is passed down from the mother. Each chromosome contains genes that provide instructions, or coding, for producing the various proteins that make up our cells. DNA stores this genetic information in its chemical structure. As genes interact, they also work together to produce phenotypes (i.e., physical traits such as eye color). Healthy individuals possess the appropriate number of chromosomes and the appropriate number of genes. When the number of chromosomes is incorrect or there are extra or defective genes, health problems occur (Amen 2017, 111). *Epigenetics* refers to factors that influence the expression of genes. Genes only account for phenotype when they are expressed and actually create proteins. Consequently, the phenotype is also dependent on environment, experience and other epigenetic influences. Because a single gene can produce several different proteins, the specific proteins produced and their associations are significantly greater than the number of genes. For instance, the APP gene, which is associated with early-onset AD, has been found to have a variant that offers protection from AD (Jonsson et al. 2012).

## Single-Nucleotide Polymorphisms

Specific genes are found on specific chromosomes in regions that code for proteins. Slight variations in one base pair in both the coding and the non-coding regions of DNA are called single-nucleotide polymorphisms (SNPs). SNPs are most often found in the non-coding areas between genes. SNPs are the most common genetic variation found in humans, and they occur in about every 1,000 nucleotides. This amounts to roughly four to five million SNPs in every person's genome.

While SNPs do not cause disease, some of these variations are associated with risk for certain diseases. SNPs that are rare, occurring in less than 1 percent of the population, are called mutations. When SNPs are common in a population, they're called polymorphisms, and when they're relatively common, they're called single-nucleotide polymorphisms. Scientists have found more than 100 million SNPs in populations throughout the world. Each human newborn has about 60 new mutations (Heine 2017, 17).

SNPs can result from copying errors when new DNA strands are replicated, and they are rarely an improvement on the original gene, although they can occur in future generations as a result of natural selection. More often, a mutated gene is detrimental and comes with a cost to the individual. In this case, the mutation decreases in future generations because those with the mutation are less likely to survive and reproduce.

Mutations can be acquired at any time in life, especially in aging individuals. It's thought that cells can only divide a limited number of times, and with age genomic instability occurs. Acquired mutations, which can be caused by DNA copying errors, radiation therapies, cellular wear and tear, ultraviolet radiation from the sun, and chemical carcinogens such as aflatoxin B1, typically occur only in certain cells, not in every cell in the body. However, these acquired or somatic mutations, when present in egg or sperm cells, can be passed on to offspring, even when the mutations are not present in other cells in the parents.

### De Novo Mutations

New mutations, which can be hereditary or acquired, are referred to as *de novo mutations*. In some cases, the mutation occurs in an egg or sperm cell but is not present in any of the individual's other cells, although the mutation can be passed on to offspring. In rare circumstances, the mutation occurs in the fertilized egg shortly after the egg and sperm cells unite. When this situation occurs, as the fertilized egg divides, the growing embryo will have the mutation in every cell, presumably as a result of the mutation occurring in stem cells. In genetic disorders that occur in a child whose parents both lack the responsible mutation, de novo mutations are the likely cause.

### Hereditability

*Hereditability* refers to how much of a trait's variance within a given sample is due to genetics. Besides eye color, body mass, height, and metabolism rates, psychological characteristics are also hereditary, including whether one believes in God, has a tendency to get divorced, likes jazz music, or is likely to get mugged (Heine 2017, 30–36).

## Genes in Early-Onset AD

In EOAD, which affects less than 5 percent of the population, signs and symptoms of AD usually appear in individuals between the ages of 30 and 65 years. EOAD is strongly linked to three specific gene mutations: presenilin 1 (PSEN1), presenilin 2 (PSEN2), or amyloid precursor protein (APP). The APOE-ε4 gene is also sometimes seen in cases of EOAD, and in some cases of EOAD, no mutations associated with AD have been found.

The APP gene on chromosome 21q is also associated with Down syndrome (trisomy 21). These patients tend to develop amyloid deposits as well as the characteristic symptoms of AD when in their 40s.

## Missense Mutations

Missense mutations are point mutations in which a single-nucleotide change results in a codon that codes for a different amino acid. Amino acids are the building blocks of proteins. Missense mutations have been identified in the APP gene on chromosome 21 at position 717 in a small number of EOAD cases. These mutations encode amino acid substitutions near or within the region encompassing the amyloid beta protein gene.

In several families with this disorder, the normal valine residue is replaced with other amino acids, including isoleucine, glycine, or phenylalanine. Cells that express mutated APP at position 717 secrete increased levels of amyloid beta 1–42 and amyloid beta 1–43, which tend to rapidly form very toxic amyloid fibrils (Kandel et al. 2000, 1156).

## Familial AD

In autosomal dominant AD or early-onset familial AD, which is responsible for less than 1 percent of all cases of AD and has been found in slightly more than 600 families worldwide, the disease is caused by a hereditary mutation to one of the three genes associated with EOAD. Inheriting one of these mutated genes from either parent typically leads to a 50 percent chance of inheriting the mutation and symptoms occurring earlier, usually between age 30 and 50. The majority of these mutations, including the Swedish and London mutations, are in or adjacent to the amyloid beta peptide sequence.

The PSEN1 gene is involved with gamma-secretase enzyme activity, intracellular signaling, and amyloid beta production. A mutation in the PSEN1 gene on chromosome 14 has been found in more than 450 families worldwide, and more than 176 mutations have been discovered (Bekris et al. 2010). This number represents about 80 percent of all cases of familial AD. Symptoms can occur as early as age 30. Presenilins are major components of aspartyl protease enzyme complexes that regulate the gamma-secretase cleavage of APP. PSEN1 mutations are thought to increase the ratio of amyloid beta 42 to amyloid beta 40, which causes a change in function, leading to reduced gamma-secretase activity. Deposits of amyloid beta 42 may represent an early preclinical event in PSEN1 mutation carriers (Bekris et al. 2010).

The PSEN2 gene is involved with gamma-secretase enzyme activity, amyloid beta production, and synaptic plasticity. More than 30 families have been found to have a mutation in the PSEN2 gene on chromosome 1 that causes a condition of familial AD that occurs later in life than that seen in individuals with the PSEN1 mutation. The age of onset is highly variable, ranging from age 45 to 88 years. Missense mutations in the PSEN2 gene are a rare cause of early-onset familial AD (at least in the Caucasian populations studied). Missense mutations in the PSEN2 gene may have lower penetrance than missense mutations in the PSEN1 gene. PSEN2 missense mutations may increase the modifying action of other genes or environmental influences.x Unlike PSEN1, the PSEN2 gene causes a reduction in amyloid beta production, although there is a significant increase in the toxic amyloid beta 42 protein (Bekris et al. 2010).

The APP gene is associated with neuronal development (including synapse formation and repair) and amyloid beta production. More than 32 missense mutations in the APP gene have been identified in 85 families. Most of these mutations are located at the secretase enzyme cleavage site or the APP transmembrane domain. Information on APP mutations is regularly updated by the National Center for Biotechnology Information and in the Alzheimer Disease Mutation Database (www.molgen.ua.ac.be/ADMutations).

More than 100 families worldwide have a mutation in the APP gene on chromosome 21 (which is also seen in Down syndrome) that causes the buildup of amyloid beta protein in the brain leading to familial AD (Alzheimer's Society 2019). More than 30 mutations have been found, 25 of which are pathogenic. In most cases, these mutations have caused autosomal dominant early-onset AD. These mutations primarily cause overproduction of amyloid beta protein, with a shift toward increased production of the toxic amyloid beta 42 protein. One of the rare variants of APP, N660Y, has also been found to cause LOAD (Jonsson et al. 2012).

While most experts do not recommend genetic testing for patients with LOAD, in EOAD genetic testing may be appropriate.

### Protective Mutations

Researchers searching for low-frequency variants in the APP gene have discovered a coding mutation (A673T) that protects against AD and cognitive decline in the normal elderly population. This mutation causes a 40 percent reduction of amyloid peptides as part of in vitro studies, and it reduces beta-secretase cleavage of APP (Jonsson et al. 2012).

## DNA Methylation

Epigenetics changes how genes are expressed without changing the genes. Methylation is an example of epigenetics. Methylation is a normal biochemical process in which a methyl group is transferred from one substance to another. In DNA methylation, which is an epigenetic mark, a methyl group is transferred from the compound S-adenosylmethionine (SAMe) to position

5 of the cytosine nucleotide on DNA, where it forms 5-methylcytosine. When a gene is methylated in this fashion, its expression is reduced.

With optimal methylation, the activity of the various bodily systems is at its best, including activities related to DNA and neurotransmitter production, histamine, fat, and estrogen metabolism, liver and eye health, detoxification, and cellular energy.

In order to have adequate SAMe, the B vitamin 5-MTHF (also known as active folate or methylfolate) must be present. However, 60 percent of the U.S. population has a genetic mutation that reduces their ability to absorb folic acid and create enough MTHF. Without adequate SAMe, the body is unable to produce adequate amounts of molecules critical to health, including glutathione, coenzyme Q10, melatonin, serotonin, nitric oxide, norepinephrine, epinephrine, L-carnitine, cysteine, and taurine (Miller 2018). Blood tests for the MTHF enzyme methylenetetrahydrofolate reductase are widely available.

In histone modification, epigenetic changes occur in histone proteins. Normally, DNA wraps around these proteins to form chromatin. Gene expression is reduced or intensified depending on how tight or loose the chromatin structure is, with looser chromatin causing greater gene expression.

Besides mutations, DNA expression can be altered by a number of environmental factors, including those that affect DNA methylation and histone modifications. These changes to DNA can be passed down to offspring. Supplements and lifestyle changes that help improve the methylation cycle and histone modification are described in Chapter Twelve.

## Genes in Late-Onset AD

While the APOE gene polymorphism has been studied the longest and appears to have the strongest association with LOAD, more than 30 small gene variants or DNA regions have now been identified by gene-wide association studies that increase or decrease the risk of a person developing AD. More new gene variants are likely to be found. All of these genes are involved in how the body responds to tissue debris that builds up in the brain after an infection or other problem (Weintraub 2019).

For this reason, human innate immune genes have emerged as the largest group of risk factors for LOAD (Moir et al. 2018). Genes that have variants associated with an intermediate increased or decreased LOAD risk include:

- ABCA7, which is involved in cholesterol metabolism
- ACE, which is involved in cell tracking, lipid transport, and the immune response
- ADAM10, which is involved in cell tracking, lipid transport, and the immune response

- ADAMTS1, which is involved in cell tracking, lipid transport, and the immune response
- BIN1, which is involved in inflammation and immunity, fat metabolism, and transport within cells
- CD2AP, which is involved in inflammation and immunity, fat metabolism, and transport within cells
- CD33, which is involved in inflammation and immunity, fat metabolism, and transport within cells
- CLU, which regulates clusterin and helps clear amyloid beta protein from the brain (also involved in cholesterol metabolism)
- CR1, which reduces production of a protein that regulates brain inflammation
- EPHA1, which is involved in inflammation and immunity, fat metabolism, and transport within cells
- IQCK, which is involved in cell tracking, lipid transport, and the immune response
- MS4A, which is involved in inflammation and immunity, fat metabolism, and transport within cells
- PICALM, which is associated with neuronal signaling
- PLD3, which is involved in inflammation and immunity, fat metabolism, and transport within cells
- SHIP1, which is involved with the immune response, with SNPs affecting microglial cells
- SORL1, which encodes a mosaic protein associated with the vacuolar protein sorting 10 (VPS10) domain-containing receptor family, as well as the low-density lipoprotein receptor (also involved in cholesterol metabolism)
- rare variants of TREM2, which is the triggering receptor expressed on myeloid cells-2, involved in the modulation of inflammatory signaling; several variants of TREM2 have found been to increase the risk of LOAD by two- to four-fold (Gratuze et al. 2018)
- WWOX, which is involved in cell tracking, lipid transport, and the immune response

## The APOE Gene

The apolipoprotein E (APOE) gene is found on chromosome 19. The protein encoded by this gene is responsible for handling the body's fats, including cholesterol. APOE is a very low-density lipoprotein that removes cholesterol from the blood and transports it to the brain and liver for processing. In the central nervous system, APOE coordinates the mobilization and redistribution of cholesterol, phospholipids, and fatty acids, which are essential for neuronal development, brain plasticity, and cellular membrane repair functions.

The polymorphisms seen in APOE are unique to humans, and it has been suggested that these polymorphisms evolved as a result of adaptive changes to diet considering that individuals with APOE-ε4 tend to have higher levels of total and LDL cholesterol. In vitro studies show that neurons have a lower cholesterol uptake when lipid molecules are bound to APOE-ε4 compared to being bound to APOE-ε2 and APOE-ε3. In addition, APOE-ε4 appears to be less efficient than the other allele forms in promoting the removal of cholesterol from neurons and astrocytes (Bekris et al. 2010).

While the APOE gene has five alleles, only three of these alleles—ε2, ε3, and ε4—show a significant association with increased or decreased AD risk. The APOE gene is associated with both familial late-onset and sporadic late-onset AD.

Because individuals inherit one allele from each parent, there are six possible combinations: ε2/ε2; ε2/ε3; ε2/ε4; ε3/ε3; ε3/ε4; and ε4/ε4. Increased risk for AD is associated with the ε4 allele. About 15 percent of the population has one ε4 allele, and, while the gene frequency varies in different ethnicities, in Caucasians only about 1–2 percent of the population has APOE-ε4/ε4. The risk of AD from APOE-ε4 is also found in African Americans and Caribbean Hispanics. In men with ε4/ε4 alleles, the risk of developing AD by age 73 is 25 percent, whereas in women with ε4/ε4, the risk of developing AD by age 73 is 45 percent (Bekris et al. 2010).

A person with one APOE-ε4 allele has 2.5 times the risk of developing AD, and someone with two copies of the ε4 allele has 5–15 times the risk of developing AD (Amen 2017, 113). Individuals with one copy of APOE-ε4 have a 75 percent chance of not developing AD. However, the risk factors for AD are slightly higher in people with the AD allele who have immediate family members with AD. The risk for AD is also higher in individuals with ε2 and ε3 alleles if they have family members with AD. The risk of developing AD increases with age regardless of one's APOE alleles.

White individuals of European ancestry with ε3/ε3 alleles have a 10–15 percent risk of developing mild cognitive impairment (MCI) related to AD by age 85. Those with the ε3/ε4 genotype have a 20–25 percent risk of developing MCI by age 85 (BAI Beacon 2017). The ε2/ε2 isoform of APOE is rarely seen, making it difficult to obtain risk ratios, although it is thought to offer protection from developing AD. The presence of the APOE-ε4 allele in other races can differ both in frequency and in its association with AD. While APOE-ε4 is more common in people of African descent, it has a smaller association with cognitive decline.

In addition, people with the APOE-ε4 allele who develop AD as a result of other causes (such as injuries to the blood-brain barrier) develop AD about two to five years earlier than people without the gene. Individuals with one or two ε4 alleles also have a greater risk for vascular disease. In individuals with central nervous system infections, the presence of the ε4 allele increases their risk of developing AD. Individuals with the APOE-ε4 allele also have higher degrees of amyloid and neurofibrillary tau tangle pathology and an increase in mitochondrial damage compared to individuals with AD who do not have the APOE-ε4 allele (Bekris et al. 2010).

## Commercial APOE Genome Testing

Most experts do not recommend testing for the APOE gene in the absence of symptoms unless one is interested in participating in a clinical trial. Apparently, it is very common for APOE-ε4 to be underrepresented by some companies that provide raw DNA data, while it is overrepresented in other reports. A caution from Promethease, a testing company that analyzes the raw data generated by Ancestry.com, 123.com and many other testing sites, alerts clients to the fact that APOE results (and several other DNA results) are likely to be incorrect. Promethease finds that in the raw DNA provided by these companies, many polymorphisms are overrepresented. Sequencing the APOE gene is difficult and subject to error.

Steven J. Heine, the distinguished university scholar and professor of social and cultural psychology at the University of British Columbia, cautions that direct-to-consumer companies that analyze DNA data are unable to provide specific predictions about health risks for common diseases because common diseases do not have a clear set of causes that can be faithfully read from one's genes. Heine is also the author of *DNA Is Not Destiny: The Remarkable, Completely Misunderstood Relationship Between You and Your Genes* (Heine 2017, 96).

## APOE-ε4 and Other Associations

APOE-ε4 is known to cause several toxic effects on the cerebrovascular system that contribute to neurodegeneration. Defects in the blood-brain barrier (BBB) related to pro-inflammatory cyclophilin A are greater in patients with the APOE-ε4 gene. APOE-ε4 has also been found to cause an age-dependent breakdown of the BBB by activating cyclophilin A in the brain's capillary pericyte cells. APOE-ε2 and APOE-ε3 genes are known to suppress the cyclophilin A pathway, with no effect on the BBB. APOE-ε4 is also known to decrease the normal clearance of amyloid beta protein from the brain (Myslinski 2014).

APOE-ε4 is associated with cardiovascular disease, deep vein thrombosis, elevated lipid levels (which increase levels of amyloid beta protein), increased reactivation of the *Herpes simplex* virus, and atherosclerosis. In contrast to its effects among the elderly, young healthy patients with APOE-ε4 are reported to have better episodic memory and neural efficiency. In a study of individuals living in low-income housing, researchers found that in APOE-ε4 carriers without MCI or AD, vitamin E levels tended to be low. In APOE-ε4 carriers with MCI, vitamin A levels tended to be low, and subjects were more likely to be obese (Shahar et al. 2013). Low levels of vitamin E have long been associated with AD.

## Genes and Microbes

Studies show that a number of brain infections, including the *Herpes simplex* virus, are more likely to be seen in AD patients with the APOE-ε4 allele (Itzhaki 2018). In addition, the brains of individuals with late-onset dementia who have the ε4 allele have been found to contain a greater number of *Chlamydia pneumoniae*–infected cells compared to individuals without the ε4 allele. This finding is consistent with the role of ε4 in enhancing the movement of *C. pneumoniae* from the pulmonary system to astroglial and microglial cells in the central nervous system (Balin et al. 2018). Lipopolysaccharides released from gram-negative bacteria are also known to cause the neuropathology seen in patients with LOAD.

## CRISPR Therapies

The prokaryotic bacteria and archae do not possess immune system cells. Instead, they use enzymes in a system called clustered regularly interspaced short palindromic repeats (CRISPR). In this system, parts of the microbial genome have sequences of DNA derived from viruses (bacteriophages) that have previously infected the prokaryote. These DNA sequences are used much like T lymphocyte cells to detect and ultimately destroy the DNA of similar viruses and bacteriophages during subsequent infections. Like the immune system's immunological memory, the CRISPR system remembers previous threats and prevents them from recurring.

Emmanuelle Charpentier at the Helmholtz Centre for Infection Research has explained that CRISPR involves the bacterial ability to capture pieces of DNA from an invading virus, storing these pieces of DNA in specific areas of their genome, converting the viral DNA copy into copies of RNA and then mobilizing the RNA pieces along with DNA-digesting enzymes to attack the DNA of the virus that dares to strike again (Dietert 2016, 239).

Techniques used to alter genes are based on CRISPR, and the genes employed for producing the DNA-cutting enzymes are called CRISPR-associated genes (Cas). The Cas enzyme seeks a precise match for the RNA that brings specificity into the attack. A particular Cas—Cas9—appears to be very important in giving the entire immune-like defense system its capacity of memory. Much like an immune response, the process targets only pathogenic viruses, although it is also selective against an autoimmune response. The CRISPR-Cas9 system overlaps with the human immune system in many ways (Dietert 2016, 240).

CRISPR-Cas9 may provide a solution to certain ailments by knocking out genes known to cause disease. But this approach raises legitimate concerns about designer babies and GMO foods. Altering genes also begs the question of whether doing so will eliminate some of our humanness (Heine 2017, 97). CRISPR-based therapies are being studied in mice as treatments for Alzheimer's disease.

## DNAm PhenoAge

Many epigenetic clocks have been developed in recent years. These clocks determine biological age and predict how long a human is likely to live, as well as their risk for AD and related neuropathologies. DNAm ("m" for methylation) PhenoAge was developed by Morgan Levine while working with Steve Horvath as a postdoctoral researcher at Harvard. DNAm PhenoAge is a tool for predicting a variety of aging outcomes, including mortality, cancers, healthspan, physical functioning and Alzheimer's disease. Here, the researchers found that an increase in epigenetic marks, relative to chronological age, is associated with increased activation of pro-inflammatory and interferon pathways and decreased transcriptional/translational machinery, DNA damage response and mitochondrial function.

With this tool, the researchers look for areas where the nucleotides cytosine and guanine are linked to a phosphate molecule. These areas are ripe for methyl groups to link to the cytosine nucleotide in specific sequences on both DNA strands. These areas of increased DNA methylation are then correlated with a number of blood markers not related to genes, such as albumin and alkaline phosphatase (markers for liver function); C-reactive protein (marker of inflammation and immune function); lymphocyte percent and white blood cell count (markers of immune function); red blood cell parameters (markers of general health); and metabolic markers such as lipid levels, glucose, insulin, and age. To calculate DNAm PhenoAge, these measures are also correlated with lifestyle, including exercise, dietary habits (particularly consumption of fruits and vegetables, which were evaluated with carotenoid levels and other nutrient levels), education, and socioeconomic status.

## DNAm PhenoAge in Alzheimer's Disease

Using postmortem data from the Religious Order Study and the Memory and Aging Project, Levine and her colleagues measured the DNAm PhenoAge in the dorsolateral prefrontal cortex of subjects with AD and age-matched controls and found the DNAm PhenoAge to be much higher in the subjects with AD, meaning that their biological age was higher than their chronological or expected age. In addition, a higher DNAm PhenoAge was seen in subjects with a higher amyloid load, more diffuse neuritic plaques, and more neurofibrillary tangles (Levine et al. 2018).

Levine explains that increased methylation causes individuals to have a higher DNAm PhenoAge than their biological age. Other epigenetic clocks, including the DNA GrimAge (after the Grim Reaper), have also demonstrated increased methylation as a result of smoking, alcohol, and exposure to particulate matter from vehicular traffic, and they can be used to predict mortality and disease risk. Levine describes these epigenetic changes as a consequence of lifestyle as well as mitochondrial dysfunction, defects in neuronal signaling, and immune system aging (Nwanaji-Enwerem et al. 2016; Hunt 2019; Mitteldorf 2019).

Epigenetic clocks continue to be explored, and researchers are finding that the maintenance of DNA methylation patterns throughout DNA replication cycles may also be mediated directly by specific environmental cues. These cues include consequences of the changing microbiome; altered immunity as a result of antibiotics; antibiotic resistance; infections (particularly in individuals receiving treatment for HIV infection); early-life environmental conditions, including inadequate fetal growth; early menopause; famine and poor nutrition; and exposure to environmental toxins (Levine et al. 2018; Vaiserman 2018).

## Summary

In the rare conditions of early-onset Alzheimer's disease, three inheritable gene mutations are known to directly cause disease, and these conditions (which represent less than 5 percent of all cases of AD) are found in a small number of families.

The APOE gene, which is involved in transporting lipids to the liver and brain, has three alleles: APOE-ε2, APOE-ε3, and APOE-ε4. The ε4 allele of APOE is a risk factor for late-onset AD, although most individuals with this allele do not develop AD. The risk of AD increases when two copies of APOE-ε4 are present and when an individual has one parent or two siblings with AD.

More than 30 other gene mutations have also been found to have slight associations with AD, and most of these genes are involved in the immune system's response to tissue debris. Lifestyle, diet, and other environmental factors may have a greater influence than genes in LOAD development.

Using CRISPR-Cas9 therapies mimics the prokaryote's response to viral threats. These therapies, which involve gene manipulation, are being investigated as potential treatment for various conditions.

Gene mutations are usually caused by copying errors and are associated with diseases, whereas epigenetic markers change the expression of genes. DNA methylation is an example of epigenetics that is associated with aging and disease risk. Epigenetic clocks are becoming increasingly accurate in predicting risk factors for mortality and disease, including AD.

# TWELVE

# Risk Reduction
# and Therapies

Regardless of one's genetic makeup, everyone is at risk for Alzheimer's disease as they grow older. However, based on the definition of dementia as a decline in cognitive abilities that leads to a loss of independence, a number of published studies show that the age-specific risk of dementia has declined over the past 40 years (Satizabal et al. 2016). Although the reasons for this decline are not clear, an increase in educational attainment and better control of cardiovascular risks such as hypertension have been suggested.

Although the incidence of diabetes has surged in recent years, improved treatments between 2000 and 2012 may have decreased dementia risk. Contributions from exercise, diet, social ties, nutritional supplements, and a reduction in smoking have also helped. In addition, an understanding of the microbiome has emerged, which has led to a better understanding of the importance of gastrointestinal health and avoiding toxins. In this chapter, the factors found to reduce the risk of AD are described, along with information on new therapies that are under investigation.

## Optimizing Neural Function

Neuronal or brain plasticity refers to the fact that neurons regenerate throughout life in a process known as neurogenesis. Neurogenesis occurs in the olfactory bulb, the subventricular zone, and the dentate gyri of the hippocampus (Crews and Masliah 2010). During this process, neurons proliferate, migrate, differentiate, grow and form synaptic connections. Neurogenesis is reported to be defective in AD. During aging and in the disease progression that occurs in AD, synaptic plasticity and the integrity of neurons are disturbed, which leads to neurodegeneration. A number of defects in signaling molecules and disruptions to cell receptors are thought to be involved in this process.

The good news is that there are a number of factors, including exercise, physiological substances (neurotrophic growth factors and peptides), gene therapies, lithium, vaccinations, and diet, that have a positive effect on brain plasticity and the generation of new neurons.

Plasticity also encompasses the concept that learning tasks that are associated with certain areas of the brain can affect nearby neurons. For instance, a common observation is that learning to play musical instruments can increase synaptic connections in neighboring brain regions affecting math concepts, thereby improving math skills.

## Brain-Derived Neurotrophic Factor (BDNF)

Brain-derived neurotrophic factor (BDNF) is a growth factor encoded by the BDNF gene on chromosome 11. Neurotrophic factors, such as BDNF and nerve growth factor, are cytokines that influence nerve growth in the brain and peripheral nervous system. BDNF helps regenerate new neurons and aids existing neurons in surviving and forming new synaptic connections. Polymorphisms to the BDNF gene can interfere with neuronal survival and neurodegeneration.

BDNF is also known to help reduce depression, improve sleep, protect against neurodegeneration and amplify weight loss. BDNF levels can increase with intermittent fasting, exercise, meditation, deep sleep, sunlight, and calorie restriction.

## Nerve Growth Factor

Nerve growth factor (NGF) was the first neurotrophic factor to be discovered. NGF has been found to play a critical protective role in the development and survival of sympathetic, sensory and forebrain cholinergic neurons. In addition, NGF promotes the outgrowth of neuronal extension, and it promotes nerve cell recovery after ischemic, surgical or chemical injuries (Aloe et al. 2015).

NGF is known to promote the healing of many tissues and cells, including the cells of the eye. A protector of the central and peripheral nervous systems, NGF promotes survival of degenerating peripheral nerve cells and assists with the maintenance and protection of neurotransmitters and neuropeptides. NGF also promotes the synthesis of sympathetic and sensory nerve cells. In neurodegenerative disorders, low levels of NGF are seen. Preparations containing NGF have been used to treat these disorders.

The first study demonstrating that NGF could be safely delivered to damaged brain neurons was published by Chen and colleagues, who showed that NGF administered via the nasal cavity can protect the damaged cholinergic neurons of the basal forebrain and improve the behavioral performance in AD experimental models (Aloe et al. 2015).

## Supplements for Brain Health

In recent years, many multi-ingredient supplements for brain health have been introduced. According to the AARP Collaborative Council in a report issued in June 2019, these products offer little value and are a waste of money, with the exception of vitamins B12 and B9 (folate) used for people with deficiencies of these nutrients (Fifield 2019). Still, according to other specialists, there are many individual nutrients that are essential for brain health and offer considerable benefits.

## Nutrient Deficiencies in Alzheimer's Disease

About 60 percent of adults in the United States have methylenetetrahydrofolate reductase mutations that cause them to absorb folate poorly. Activated methylated forms of folate are required for these individuals to have adequate folate. Deficiencies of folate and vitamin B12 can both cause conditions of dementia.

Low levels of these vitamins also cause an increase in plasma homocysteine levels. Even levels slightly above the homocysteine reference range can dramatically increase the risk of AD. By reducing inflammation and improving homocysteine levels, folate can enhance cognitive performance. Folate is also able to modify gene expression. Without adequate folate, genes involved in producing amyloid beta are turned on (Ma et al. 2017).

Patients with AD are known to have low levels of 25-OH vitamin D and vitamin E. Researchers have found that certain cells in the brain have receptors for vitamins D and E that help the brain carry out its normal functions. Vitamin D3 has been shown to support neurogenesis and protect against neuroinflammation. Higher levels of vitamin D are associated with improved recovery and reduced cognitive impairment following strokes.

Many people have low levels of vitamin E, and low levels are a well-known cause of dementia. Vitamin E was first proposed as a treatment for AD many years ago. Because not everyone with AD has a vitamin E deficiency, it has been difficult to assess the benefits of treatment. However, the levels of vitamin E in patients with AD are lower than the levels seen in non-demented controls.

Vitamin E is an antioxidant, and it is known to enhance the immune response in elderly people. However, more studies are needed before the effectiveness of vitamin E in AD can be fully ascertained (Lioret et al. 2019).

The amino acid taurine is also known to facilitate recovery in both ischemic and hemorrhagic stroke, and it reduces the effects of neurotoxins. In addition, taurine helps promote neurogenesis and reduces the effects of oxidative stress (Rak et al. 2014).

Daniel Amen recommends a number of herbs for their ability to improve memory, learning and other brain functions. In particular, he recommends saffron, *Bacopa monnieri*, and sage (Amen 2017, 92–3). Sage has long been known to improve attention and prevent age-related cognitive decline. Amen also recommends avoiding sugar and foods that turn to sugar and limiting consumption of charred meats, cigarette smoke, and car exhaust.

For reducing the risk of AD, the Life Extension Foundation recommends wild blueberry extract, curcumin, pregnenolone, ashwaganda extract, and sage extract, and placebo-controlled trials show that lithium treatment may also benefit patients with AD (Life Extension Staff 2018).

## Iron and the Brain

The geneticist Preston Estep finds that the brain is damaged by the typical iron levels recommended as standard dietary intakes. Iron accumulates over time and accumulates in areas of the brain associated with age-dependent neurodegeneration. In their younger years, women are protected against iron excess through menstruation, but after menopause iron tends to accumulate.

Although iron deficiency was once a big problem in the United States, those days are long gone. Due to fortification programs, iron excess is now a greater issue. Estep writes that countries that lead the world in physical and mental health eat large amounts of nonfortified, refined grain products (Estep 2016).

In his "Mindspan Diet," Estep advocates a Mediterranean-style diet and an avoidance of foods high in iron content. Because iron has long been a risk factor for AD, and the measure of ferritin levels is one of the main screening tests used to rule out other causes of dementia, Estep's plan offers many benefits. Other foods that make up the Mediterranean diet, such as white rice and olive oil, help patients handle carbohydrates without the glucose spikes that occur in the traditional American diet.

## Resilience and Cognitive Reserve

*Superagers* is a term used to describe individuals who age exceptionally well and retain good cognitive function. These individuals are reported as being either resistors or resilient. As resistors, they avoid the usual maladies of aging such as cardiac disease. As resilient, they have survived disease or other personal setbacks with a high level of function, bouncing back gracefully. Superagers do not typically have AD even when they experience the neuropathological changes of AD.

Cognitive reserve has been found to reduce the likelihood of developing AD. Cognitive reserve is related to either the brain's anatomical reserves (which allow them to tolerate neuropathology) or an individual's resilience.

The risk of AD is also reduced in people who grow up bilingual, have advanced educations and/or challenging jobs, remain active in old age, and have meaningful social contacts.

## Diet, Exercise, and Brain Health

Following a healthy diet reduces inflammation and the risks of neurodegeneration. Dr. David Perlmutter explains that through diet we can spark epigenetic changes that increase neurogenesis and fortify existing brain circuits with entirely new and elaborate connections (Perlmutter 2013, 128).

Because of the toxic effects of refined grains on brain health, adopting a grain-free diet is one of the best dietary changes an individual can make. Because grains cause an increase in blood glucose, avoiding grains also helps prevent glucose spikes, type 2 diabetes and inflammation. Dr. Perlmutter recommends a ketogenic diet for brain health and the addition of the dietary supplements: DHA, resveratrol, turmeric (curcumin), probiotics, alpha lipoic acid, coconut oil, bioactive B vitamins, vitamin E, and vitamin D (Perlmutter 2013, 186–192).

Low levels of omega-3 fatty acids are seen in AD. In particular, low levels of the omega-3 fatty acids EPA and DHA are associated with inflammation, heart disease, depression, obesity, cognitive impairment and dementia (Amen 2017, 92). Supplements containing DHA and EPA are reported to enhance brain health. The Omega-3 Index is a blood test that measures the total amounts of EPA and DHA. A low Omega-3 Index level increases the risk of cognitive decline by as much as 77 percent. The goal is to aim for an Omega-3 Index level higher than 8 percent.

The antioxidant dietary supplement alpha lipoic acid (ALA) has been found to improve brain health in AD patients. ALA is known to activate an enzyme that facilitates increased production of the neurotransmitter acetylcholine while simultaneously increasing the availability of glucose for use by neurons in the brain.

Researchers at Johns Hopkins University School of Medicine teamed up with researchers at the National Institute on Aging to identify core mechanisms that contribute to AD. Their findings indicate that the NAD$^+$ precursor nicotinamide riboside is able to restore brain plasticity, allowing neurons to store memory. In a mouse model closely resembling AD, the researchers found that supplementing with nicotinamide riboside improved cognitive function. Recent evidence indicates that defective DNA repair mechanisms are a primary contributor to the development of AD. $NAD^+$ is a cellular metabolite that is essential for mitochondrial health and biogenesis, stem cell self-renewal, and neuronal stress resistance. Boosting $NAD^+$ has been found to improve DNA repair and reduce the number of toxic P-tau proteins in animal models of AD (Hou et al. 2018).

Exercise is important for neurogenesis because it boosts BDNF levels. A study from Rush University's Memory and Aging Project showed that individuals in the lowest percentile of daily physical activity had a 230 percent greater risk of developing AD compared to those in the highest percentiles of physical activity (Perlmutter 2013, 203).

## Optimizing Immune Function

The main diseases associated with aging, such as dementia, cancer, and pneumonia, are all linked to an ineffective immune system. In immunosenescence (the immune system's age-associated decline), failing cells create a state of hyperinflammation that destroys neurons and allows cancer cells to grow. More than 70 percent of the human immune system resides in the gut. Here, microbes keep yeast in check and protect us from other harmful microorganisms by launching an immune response when they encounter pathogens.

Having an intact intestinal barrier is key to preventing the escape of microbes. Avoiding toxins, having a steady supply of essential nutrients, taking prebiotics and probiotics, and following an active lifestyle all help to strengthen the immune system.

Vaccines can help because they boost the immune system's production of antibodies and strengthen the immune response. Studies show that elderly people who receive an annual influenza vaccine are less likely to develop AD.

### Nutrients for Immune System Health

Researchers have identified three natural compounds that can reverse the harmful changes that occur in the aged immune system. These three compounds are extracts of reishi mushrooms, cistanche and pu-erh tea. Extracts of these compounds have been found to increase the production of both T lymphocytes and natural killer cells while lowering levels of the pro-inflammatory cytokines interleukin-6 and TNF-alpha.

The nutrient-rich Mediterranean diet, which contains minimal amounts of processed foods, is also recommended for immune system health because it is associated with protection from inflammation and oxidative stress. The Mediterranean diet consists of high intakes of whole grains, legumes, fresh vegetables, fruit, extra-virgin olive oil, nuts and seeds, moderate amounts of fish, and small amounts of dairy products and wine. Low levels of magnesium and fiber, both of which are abundant in the Mediterranean diet, have been linked to inflammation and are known to cause an elevated C-reactive-protein level.

A team of international researchers has investigated the immune system processes that lead to AD and worked to discover natural compounds that improve these and other signaling processes. They listed the processes that lead to neuroinflammation and neurodegeneration in AD as increased microglial activation, expression of cytokines, reactive oxygen species, and nuclear factor kappa beta (Shal et al. 2018).

The researchers write that natural polyphenolic phytochemicals have recently gained greater attention as alternative therapeutic agents against AD and are considered less toxic and more efficacious than novel synthetic drugs.

Because *Ginkgo biloba*, quercetin, and epigallocatechin-3-gallate are able to penetrate the blood-brain barrier, these flavonoids are able to directly affect the areas of the brain with high levels of inflammation in AD. Various steroid phytochemicals, such as diosgenin and prosapogenin II, have been found to have neuroprotective effects and are listed as potential therapeutic candidates for AD.

Other plant compounds with anti-inflammatory properties that are being investigated in AD include resveratrol; apigenin derivatives such as *Passiflora edulis* (passionflower); alpha-mangostin (*Garcinia mangostana*), also known as mangosteen; *Melissa officinalis* (lemon balm); *Pimpinella brachycarpa*, a member of the Family *Umbelliferae*; *Curcuma longa* (curcumin); *Zingiber officinale* (ginger); naringenin, a flavonoid found in citrus fruits; Ligraminol E4-o-beta-D-xyloside, commonly called needle fir or Manchurian fir; Panax ginseng; liminoids such as *Melia toosendan*, a family with antibacterial, neuroprotective effects and anti-cancer properties; berberine; Huperzine A; galantamine; and sophocarpidine, which is known to alleviate injury to mitochondria in neurons (Shal et al. 2018).

## Exercise and Inflammation

A number of studies involving young adults show that chronic exercise enhances immunity. A team of researchers from Qatar, Australia, Italy, England, and Switzerland conducted a study to evaluate the benefits of exercise on older individuals. They found that the most impressive changes were demonstrated by increased NK lymphocytic cells as well as increases in the general proliferation of immune cells, which is contrary to what is seen in advanced age.

## Improving Mitochondrial Function

Mitochondria are the cells' energy producers. Mitochondrial dysfunction occurs when mitochondria numbers fall too low, when defects in the mitochondrial membrane occur, when alterations in the electron transport chain occur, or when there is a lack of critical nutrient metabolites for mitochondria. These changes result in reduced energy production. Clinical trials have shown the utility of dietary supplements in restoring mitochondrial dysfunction, a condition that leads to neurodegenerative diseases such as AD (Nicolson 2014).

Nutritional supplements used to treat mitochondrial dysfunction include:

- vitamins C, D, E, B1 and B2
- minerals such as magnesium, calcium and phosphate
- membrane lipids and unsaturated fatty acids
- the metabolites creatine and pyruvate
- the cofactors CoQ10 (ubiquinone), alpha lipoic acid, NADH, and nicotinic acid
- the transporter L-carnitine, which increases the rate of mitochondrial phosphorylation that occurs in aging (also effective in sepsis and diabetes)
- the antioxidants CoQ10, alpha lipoic acid, NADH and glutathione (which can be converted from N-acetyl cysteine)
- the herbal supplements curcumin and schisandrin (Nicolson 2014)

In studies, CoQ10 (also known as ubiquinone) was shown to delay brain atrophy and amyloid beta (Aβ) plaque deposits. Administered with vitamins C and E and alpha lipoic acid, CoQ was found to reduce oxidative stress markers in patients with AD, but there were no alterations in Aβ or tau protein pathology (Nicolson 2014).

It's known that mitochondrial DNA lacks the protection afforded to nuclear DNA and consequently is damaged more by free radicals. In theories of aging, mitochondrial assault by free radicals destroys the cell from within while generating more toxic free radicals in the process. These free radicals can be broken down by a natural enzyme called superoxide dismutase, which declines with age. An absence or reduction of this enzyme is linked to AD (Kaufmann 2017, 40).

## Improving Vascular Health

Hypertension and smoking are risk factors for vascular disease. Reducing risk factors can improve vascular health. Significant vascular burden is defined as many lacunae, strategic infarcts, more than 25 percent of white matter lesions, or a combination of these characteristics. Some vascular change is typical in older populations free of dementia, suggesting that it is the degree or burden of vascular change that contributes to dementia (Livingston et al. 2017).

Studies show that epigallocatechin-3-gallate in green tea can help dissolve atherosclerotic plaques. This phytochemical is currently being studied for its ability to reduce amyloid plaques in the brain of patients with AD (Townsend et al. 2018).

## DNA Protection

Harvard University's Rudolph E. Tanzi and Lars Bertram describe AD as a "complex and genetically heterogeneous disorder that is best explained by an age-dependent dichotomous model." AD is complex because there is no single or simple mode of inheritance that can account for is heritability. AD is heterogeneous because mutations and polymorphisms in multiple genes are involved together with nongenetic factors. AD is dichotomous because the mutations in early-onset familial AD are rare, highly penetrant and transmitted in an autosomal fashion, although increased risk for late-onset AD is conferred by common polymorphisms with low penetrance but high prevalence. The complexity is greater still because the genetics in AD are currently ill defined and it is difficult to associate the gene-to-environment interactions (Tanzi and Bertram 2001).

While gene mutations can result from environmental influences such as radiation and toxins, it is important to protect DNA from additional damage. Furthermore, epigenetics provides a tool for modifying gene expression. Other modifying factors include telomeres, mediator genes, AMP kinase, mTOR, and the sirtuin gene family. Because many medications and supplements used for AD target these factors, a description of their functions is included in the following sections.

### Telomeres

Telomeres are found on the ends of DNA and are not responsible for coding proteins. Formerly considered useless, telomeres are now recognized as having an association with lifespan (depending on their length). With age, telomeres become shorter as the body's somatic cells divide and the cells' DNA is replicated. Short telomeres are somewhat associated with a shorter lifespan.

Telomerase is an enzyme with the ability to lengthen telomeres in certain cells by adding guanine sequences near the ends of DNA strands. Most human cells divide 50–70, which limits the activity of telomerase. However, in tumor cells where DNA continues to replicate, limiting telomerase offers benefits.

The immune system in elderly people weakens and becomes ineffective with age, which leads to a higher risk of infection as well as chronic inflammation and neurodegeneration. Reducing risk in AD is associated with increasing telomerase. While telomerase levels decline with age, they remain high in stem cells. Telomerase activity can be improved through lifestyle factors such as physical exercise, diet (particularly calorie restriction), dietary supplements, meditation and yoga (Kaufmann 2017, 110).

## Sirtuins

Sirtuins (silent information regulators) are genes (i.e., SIRT) and proteins (i.e., SIRT1) involved in the production of nicotinamide adenine dinucleotide (NAD)–dependent enzymes with the ability to sense environmental and nutritional stressors such as calorie restriction, oxidative stress or DNA damage. When activated, sirtuins trigger the transcription of specific proteins that boost metabolic efficiency, increase antioxidant pathways and repair DNA. Sirtuins have been found to promote longevity in most living organisms. High sirtuin levels can decrease the incidence of many inflammatory diseases, including cardiovascular disease, cancer, and type II diabetes (Kaufmann 2017, 45).

Many sirtuins are epigenetic regulators, modifying DNA or histones and assisting (along with NAD) with DNA repair mechanisms. Sirtuins also help regulate the immune system and reduce chronic inflammation. SIRT1 triggers AMP kinase, and both SIRT1 and SIRT6 inhibit the nuclear factor kappa-beta system. Increased expression of SIRT3 proteins in the elderly helps maintain healthy mitochondria and reduces the effects of aging, including increased adipose tissue (Kaufmann 2017, 60–61).

## AMP Kinase

Adenosine monophosphate-activated protein kinase (AMP kinase) is an enzyme that regulates a number of metabolic processes and initiates a signaling pathway that leads to increased energy production when it detects low levels of ATP. The end result is the breakdown of fats and glucose molecules for energy, the destruction of defective mitochondria, and the production of new mitochondria. AMP kinase is encoded by three genes, and the diabetes drug metformin is known to increase AMP kinase production.

## mTOR

The mTOR pathway is critical for early growth and development but isn't essential in later life. mTOR was found rather serendipitously when scientists discovered a new anti-fungal agent with immunosuppressant properties on Rapa Nui (also known as Easter Island) in the 1970s. Named after the location of its discovery, rapamycin has been found to target a certain signaling pathway called the "mammalian or mechanistic target of rapamycin," or mTOR. The leader of this pathway, mTOR, is a kinase enzyme in the mediator family. Like other pathway enzymes, mTOR reacts to changes in the environment such as low oxygen levels, insulin, energy status and growth factors, and it orders the biosynthesis of necessary proteins, lipids and organelles. Elderly individuals don't react well to this increased production, particularly the production of pro-inflammatory cytokines or increased resistance to hormones (Kaufmann 2017, 62).

### RAPAMYCIN

Rapamycin is used to block mTOR to counter some of the effects of aging, and it has been found to increase longevity. However, the drug has some adverse side effects due to its immunosuppressive properties, including an increased risk of infection, loss of testicular function in males, increased blood lipids, and glucose intolerance.

Both rapamycin (Sirolimus) and the related compound Everolimus suppress cellular senescence. In doing so, they can prevent age-related diseases such as atherosclerosis, obesity and neurodegeneration as they potentially rejuvenate stem cells, immunity and metabolism, especially when combined with other drugs such as metformin and lisinopril (Blagosklonny 2017).

Because AD is considered a disease of accelerated aging with a clear association with infection, a number of researchers have suggested that rapamycin be the focus of clinical trials. Currently, rapamycin is being used off-label in patients with the APOE-ε4 allele (Green 2018; Kaeberlein and Galvan 2019).

## Optimizing the Microbiome

A lack of diversity and a higher likelihood of pathogenic microorganisms are common features in the gut microbiomes of AD patients. The gut microbiome can be altered and improved through the judicious implementation of prebiotics and changes to diet, particularly adding increased amounts of fiber and fermented foods and reduced amounts of sugar, along with using alkaline water and avoiding toxins (including non-steroidal anti-inflammatory drugs and glyphosate).

With sophisticated laboratory techniques, the presence of microbes in the brains of AD patients as well as normal elderly subjects is turning out to be a common finding, although the microbiota found in the brains of AD patients is about four-fold greater. Dysbiosis in the brain microbiome is now suspected of contributing to AD. Prebiotics are non-digestible compounds in certain foods that act like fertilizers, promoting the growth and metabolism of beneficial gut microorganisms. Prebiotic fiber is fermented when it reaches the large colon. This fermentation process feeds beneficial bacterial colonies (natural gut inhabitants and probiotics) and helps to increase the number and variety of desirable bacteria in the gut. Prebiotics include apple skins, Jerusalem artichokes, onions, garlic, bananas, and chicory. The prebiotic galacto-oligosaccharide (GOS) has been studied and found to greatly reduce the neuroendocrine stress response as well as social anxiety and changes in focus and attention. GOS is now being added to some infant formulas.

Probiotics are preparations of friendly gut bacteria used to alter the gut's microbiota. Probiotics easily incorporated into one's diet include sauerkraut, kimchi, kombucha, miso, pickled herrings, soy sauce, sourdough bread, yogurt and tempeh.

While probiotics work well in altering the gut microbiome, some microbial strains produce histamines. People with histamine intolerance can exhibit symptoms when histamine levels rise. Histamine intolerance can also occur in individuals with low amounts of diamine oxidase, an enzyme that breaks histamine down. Symptoms of histamine intolerance include migraines, nasal congestion, fatigue, hives, nausea and vomiting; in more severe cases, individuals can experience abdominal cramping, tissue swelling, irregular heart rate, hypertension, anxiety, difficulty regulating body temperature and dizziness. While most people won't have problems with histamines, it's something to watch for. Probiotics with strains that don't produce histamines are available.

Fecal microbiota transplantation (FMT), which is a common therapy for patients with *Clostridium difficile* infection that doesn't respond to antibiotics, involves the transfer of stool from a carefully screened, healthy stool donor into the colon of the patient, frequently during a colonoscopy procedure. Still under investigation, FMT is used for other conditions, including multiple sclerosis and Crohn's disease. Although not yet used in AD, it may be a promising therapy for patients with this and other neurodegenerative diseases.

## Anti-Aging Supplements in AD

Anti-aging supplements are used to help prevent AD, to correct known deficiencies, to combat reactive oxygen species, to improve the microbiome and metabolic pathways, to protect against DNA mutations, and to optimize mitochondrial function. Sandra Kaufmann, MD, recommends the following supplements:

Resveratrol is fat soluble, which gives it the ability to enter cells quickly. However, it is not absorbed as well as its chemical cousin pterostilbene, which has similar properties. Both of these antioxidants enhance telomere length, have anti-inflammatory properties, activate the SIRT gene and AMP kinase, and indirectly activate DNA repair mechanisms. In animal models, resveratrol has been found to increase neuronal extensions and improve memory (Kaufmann 2017, 141–43).

Astaxanthin, which is derived from algae, is a xanthophyll carotenoid known for its red pigment, which is responsible for the bright coloring in lobsters and red crabs. As an antioxidant with powers 65 times greater than those of vitamin C, astaxanthin enhances immune system function, inhibits lipid peroxidation, regulates gene expression, improves mitochondrial function, and benefits the eyes and skin (Kaufmann 2017, 169–71).

NAD, which is converted from niacin (a form of vitamin B3), is a natural substance that declines with age. Deficiencies of vitamin B3, and subsequently NAD, cause the disease pellagra, which leads to diarrhea, dermatitis, dementia and death. NAD facilitates DNA repair and acts as a cofactor for SIRT genes and sirtuins, thereby increasing the body's energy stores.

Curcumin is an active compound found in the spice turmeric, which is derived from the roots or rhizomes of *Curcuma longa*. Curcumin has antiviral, antioxidant and anti-inflammatory properties. Due to these properties, curcumin offers benefits in neurodegenerative conditions. Curcumin has epigenetic properties and primarily affects histone acetylation. In its role as an antioxidant and free radical scavenger, it enhances the production of other antioxidant enzymes, including superoxide dismutase, and several enzymes necessary for the production of glutathione.

Carnosine is an antioxidant known for its ability to prevent the production of advanced glycation end products, which result from the same reactions that cause rubber to harden and crack. Carnosine is also known to stabilize telomere length and protect mitochondria. In addition, carnosine protects neurons both inside and outside of the brain and guards against ear damage. Because of its ability to stop the crystalline aggregation that causes eye cataracts, eye drops containing N-acetyl-carnosine are used to prevent cataracts.

The astragalus herb has long been used to protect telomeres and increase their length. Supplements are widely used as anti-aging compounds. Astragalus also has antibacterial and antiviral properties and is used to modulate the immune system.

## New Investigational Therapies

Other promising therapies include the use of bacteriophages and prions, the use of alkaline water, the use of lithium, the role of L-serine in AD and ALS, and the therapeutic use of cannabinoids.

### Bacteriophages and Prions

Amyloid proteins are prion proteins, and these proteins have been found in bacteria in yeasts. Here, prion proteins play important roles in molecular transport, secretion, cell wall development and other metabolic processes. Bacteriophages (phages) are viruses that infect specific bacteria. The role of prions in bacteriophages has not yet been examined, although bacteriophages play an important role in AD. Bacteriophages can be manipulated to target specific microbes, ones that are often resistant to antimicrobial agents. Discovered in 1915, phages were widely used to treat dysentery and cholera successfully, using phages isolated from the stools of patients who recovered from these diseases (Srisuknimit 2018). However, with the discovery of antibiotics, the use of bacteriophages was put on the back burner.

Today, these natural enemies of bacteria are once again entering the therapeutic arena. Phages inject their DNA into bacteria that they target. This DNA copies itself, makes more of the phage's shell, and packages this new DNA into a new shell. Then the phage produces toxic chemicals that rupture the bacterial host from the inside out, releasing the newly replicated phages to the outside to infect more bacteria. Because phages are specific to the bacterial species that they target, there are no alterations to the microbiome. Of greater importance, phages are able to destroy the bacterial cell walls of antibiotic-resistant bacteria (Srisuknimit 2018; Tetz and Tetz 2018).

### Alkaline Water

While tap water normally has a pH of 6–7, alkaline water has a pH of 7.5–10, which is reported to reduce reactive oxygen species, a common cause of inflammation. A number of benefits from alkaline water have been observed in patients with diabetes. The theory is that the active hydrogen molecules act much like superoxide dismutase, preventing DNA damage caused by reactive oxygen species. A Japanese study of alkaline water (used for drinking) conducted on 100 patients with senile dementia showed a slight reduction in the white blood cell count and in liver enzymes after two months. While this study observed no cognitive benefits in patients with dementia, it showed that there were no adverse effects, indicating that longer studies may be needed before cognitive improvement is seen (Yang et al. 2007).

## Paul Cox and L-serine

Paul Cox is a Harvard-trained ethnobotanist who studies indigenous people and investigates their use of native plants. Cox's interest in neurodegenerative diseases began when he set out to learn why an extraordinary number of the Chamorro people of Guam developed a disease called lytico-bodig, resembling both AD and amyotrophic lateral sclerosis (ALS). Cox eventually discovered that these Guam natives had been poisoning themselves by eating entire bats (flying fox bats) boiled in milk. This led to the discovery of a toxin called BMAA found in the cycad trees that the bats fed on.

In his Brain Chemistry Labs in Jackson, Wyoming, Cox and a group of like-minded academic researchers discovered that the cycad trees are nourished by aerial roots loaded with cyanobacteria, the oldest organism on earth (and the organism suspected of being the origin of human mitochondria). Cyanobacteria (which are referred to as blue-green algae) are ubiquitous, residing in oceans, lakes, ponds and puddles and even beneath the crust of deserts throughout the world. They are also the source of the BMAA that Cox discovered was poisoning the elderly people in Guam.

Cox and his team then began to investigate how BMAA damaged the brain. He thought that it insinuated itself into protein chains in place of one of the 20 standard amino acids. He suspected glutamate. However, a colleague found that BMAA impersonated the amino acid L-serine, causing a protein misfolding that destroyed neurons. Treatment with L-serine, a harmless amino acid, prevents BMAA's intrusion and is now being tested in clinical trials as a potential treatment for both ALS and AD (Tetzeli 2019). The trial of L-serine in AD can be found at https://clinicaltrials.gov (the clinical study identifier is NCT03062449).

## Cannabinoids

Cannabis plants contain more than 100 cannabinoid phytochemicals, but the one of most interest in AD is tetrahydrocannabinol (THC). In 2016, David Schubert and his team at the Salk Institute reported that they had found preliminary evidence that THC and other phytochemicals found in cannabis can reduce inflammation and promote the cellular removal of Aβ protein in AD (Crew 2018). This discovery supports the results of earlier studies that found evidence of the protective effects of cannabinoids, including THC, on patients with neurodegenerative disease.

Neurons have receptors for endocannabinoids, a class of endogenous lipid molecules used for intercellular signaling in the brain through the endocannabinoid receptor system. The major cannabinoid receptors are CB1 and CB2. With properties similar to the body's natural endocannabinoids, THC is able to activate these receptors. THC has been found to be the most potent CB1 agonist (able to activate the receptor). In this way, THC offers protection, removes intraneuronal Aβ and completely eliminates the production of toxic compounds. Japanese researchers have found that neuronal cell death can only be completely prevented by cannabinoids, caspase enzyme inhibitors, and lipoxygenase inhibitors. Early intervention with these compounds reduces Aβ toxicity and may reduce AD disease or progression (Currais et al. 2016).

Cannabidiol (CBD) is one of the major phytochemicals in the cannabis plant. It has proven to be very effective for treating a number of conditions, including seizure disorders. CBD directly reduces Aβ production by interacting with the amyloid precursor protein (APP). CBD modifies APP, reducing its protein levels, which results in an increased survival of neurons. Although CBD does not directly react with the endocannabinoid receptor system, it directly activates the peroxisome proliferator-activated-receptor-gamma. In doing so, CBD exerts some of its neuroprotective effects. Researchers have also found that CBD stimulates neurogenesis in the hippocampal regions of the brain. In several studies, CBD, which has no psychoactive properties, has been found to stimulate brain tissue in AD (Dach et al. 2015; Dementia Care Central 2019).

## Clinical Trials

A complete list of clinical trials can be found at https://clinicaltrials.gov. In June 2019, a search for clinical trials in AD brought up 2,140 trials at locations throughout the world. One of the largest trials involves inhibition of BACE1 (which is described in the following section), followed by several trials involved in the investigation of antimicrobial agents in AD.

### BACE1 Trials

The β-Site Amyloid Precursor Protein Cleaving Enzyme 1 (BACE1) is an enzyme required for the production of Aβ in one of the main signaling pathways leading to AD. Excessive production of BACE1 leads to Aβ protein, which is produced by neurons and other cells. As a way of reducing Aβ, several clinical trials for BACE1 inhibitors have been in the works in recent years, with some trials suspended due to a lack of results. Iqra Farooq explains that completely blocking the activity of BACE1, which produces amyloid plaques, interferes in the regulation of new neurons generated in the adult hippocampus (Farooq 2018).

Clinical trial CCNP520A2202J, "A Study of CNP520 Versus Placebo in Participants at Risk for the Onset of Clinical Symptoms of Alzheimer's Disease" (The Generations 2 Study), is currently recruiting subjects. Because earlier studies focused on patients with dementia, this trial, sponsored by Novartis, is focusing on individuals with the APOE-ε4 allele who have amyloid plaque deposits (results obtained from either cerebrospinal fluid analysis or PET scan) but have no signs of cognitive impairment based on the Mini-Mental Status Examination. This trial is scheduled to last through 2025.

## Lithium

In the 1980s, researchers from the University of Birmingham showed that lithium in 5–30 nmol/L concentrations inhibits replication of the *Herpes simplex* virus. These researchers suggested that inhibition was a result of a blockage of synthesis of viral DNA by lithium or competition with magnesium ions interfering with enzyme reactions necessary for viral replication. In a Polish-American study carried out on 69 patients with genital herpes, the general decrease of recurrence frequency was 64 percent. These results were improved further with higher concentrations of lithium.

In recent years, lithium has been studied for its possible effect on pathogenic changes in AD. The effects of lithium in these studies are attributed to inhibition of glycogen synthase kinase-3. This enzyme is essential for the metabolism of APP and the phosphorylation of tau protein (Rybakowski 2019). Additional studies have shown a lower frequency of dementia in individuals exposed to high concentrations of lithium in drinking water (Rybakowski 2019).

## Infection and Antimicrobial-Related AD Trials

In an article in a series on how Harvard researchers are tackling the issues of aging, Robert Moir commented that Alzheimer's may be a dysbiosis of the brain—a sign that the microbiome is out of whack. Rudolph Tanzi replied that if it turns out microbial culprits are identified as the cause of AD, it might be possible to treat those infections early in life, possibly with a vaccine before the earliest plaques begin to form (Powell 2017).

Tanzi believes that in many cases of AD, microbes are likely the initial seed that sets off a "toxic tumble of molecular dominoes" (Stetka 2018). Early on in the disease process, amyloid protein builds up to curb the infection, and in the process high levels of amyloid begin to impair the function of neurons in the brain. Excess amyloid then causes another protein—tau—to form tangles, which also harm neurons. Tanzi explains that the ultimate neurologic problem in AD is the body's natural reaction to this neurotoxic mess. The resulting inflammation is responsible for most of the damage in the AD brain. Tanzi speculates that in the future people could be screened at age 50, and if their brains show signs of amyloid, they will be able to knock it down a bit with antiviral medications, rather like using statins to reduce (not abolish) all cholesterol (Stetka 2018).

In July 2018, the Infectious Diseases Society of America, in collaboration with Noris, announced that it plans to offer two $50,000 grants supporting research into a microbial association with Alzheimer's. Noris reports that this is the first acknowledgment by a leading infectious disease group that AD may be microbial in nature (Stetka 2018).

## Clinical Trials on Infection in AD

Clinical trial NCT03282916, "Antiviral Therapy in Alzheimer's Disease," started in February 2018 and is still recruiting in 2019.The trial is set to last through August 2022. Sponsored by the New York State Psychiatric Institute, its collaborators are the National Institutes of Health and the National Institute on Aging. This is a placebo-matched trial using valacyclovir at 2–4 grams/day in people with *Herpes simplex* virus-1 or *Herpes simplex* virus-2. This innovative Phase II proof-of-concept trial has exceptionally high reward potential for the treatment of AD. For more information, see https://clinical-trials.gov/ct2/show/NCT03282916.

Clinical trial NCT03856359, "Trial of Rifaximin in Probably Alzheimer's Disease," is sponsored by Duke University in collaboration with Bausch Health Americas, Inc. This study aims to improve cognition and function in patients with AD by administering the oral antibiotic rifaximin. Rifaximin is a virtually non-absorbed antibiotic with the unique properties of lowering blood ammonia levels and altering gut microbiota. Ammonia levels are high in liver disease, particularly in individuals with hepatic encephalopathy. Rifaximin achieves this result by blocking bacterial RNA synthesis by increasing small bowel glutaminase. The investigators hypothesize that rifaximin will improve cognition and function in AD patients by lowering circulatory pro-inflammatory cytokines secreted by pathogenic gut bacteria. This trial is recruiting patients with middle-stage AD. For more information, see https://clinicaltrials.gov/ct2/show/NCT03856359.

Clinical trial NCT02997982, "Feasibility and Effects of Valaciclovir Treatment in Persons with Early Alzheimer's Disease" (VALZ-Pilot), sponsored by the world-renowned Alzheimer's disease researcher Hugo Lövheim, is investigating the use of the antiviral medicine valaciclovir (valacyclovir) in subjects with mild cognitive impairment or early AD. For more information, see clinicaltrials.gov/ct2/show/NCT02997982.

Even without participating in a trial, the information provided by these investigations is well worth pursuing. Many more clinical trials are focusing on infection, and a large number have local testing locations.

## Summary

This chapter describes the many factors that reduce the risk of developing AD. It's clear that in late-onset AD, environmental influences are more important than genetic risk factors. A description of the various pathways that accompany aging and the development of AD is provided. The nutritional substances described are accompanied by explanations of their physiological benefits.

This chapter also includes a discussion of clinical trials, with a focus on trials that are exploring the use of antimicrobial agents for the treatment of Alzheimer's disease.

# Bibliography

Acuña-Hinrichsen, Francisca, et al. 2019. "Herpes Simplex Virus Type 1 Enhances Expression of the Synaptic Protein Arc for Its Own Benefit." *Frontiers in Cellular Neuroscience* 12, no. 505 (January). doi:10.3389/fncel.2018.00505.

Adam, Berit, et al. 2001. "Mixed Species Biofilms of *Candida albicans* and *Staphylococcus epidermidis*." *Journal of Medical Microbiology* 51, no. 4 (April): 344–49. doi:10.109 9/0022-1317-51-4-344.

Adinolfi, Luigi, et al. 2015. "Chronic Hepatitis C Virus Infection and Neurological and Psychiatric Disorders: An Overview." *World Journal of Gastroenterology* 21, no. 8 (28 February): 2269–80. doi:10.3748/wjg.v21.i8.2269.

Aloe, Luigi, et al. 2015. "Nerve Growth Factor: A Focus on Neuroscience and Therapy." *Current Neuropharmacology* 13, no. 3 (May): 294–303. doi:10.2174/1570159X13666150403231920.

Alonso, Ruth, et al. 2018. "Infection of Fungi and Bacteria in Brain Tissue from Elderly Persons and Patients with Alzheimer's Disease." *Frontiers in Aging Neuroscience* (24 May). doi:10.3389/fnagi.2018.00159.

Alzforum: Networking for a Cure. 2018. "Aberrant Networks in Alzheimer's Tied to Herpes Viruses." 21 June. https://www.alzforum.org/news/research-news/aberrant-networks-alzheimers-tied-herpes-viruses.

Alzheimer's Association. 2018. "Advances Along the Gut-Liver-Brain Axis in Alzheimer's Disease: Why Diet May Be So Impactful." *AAIC18: The Alzheimer's Association International Conference*, 24 July. https://www.alz.org/aaic/releases_2018/AAIC18-Tues-gut-liver-brain-axis.asp.

Alzheimer's Society. 2019. "Alzheimer's Disease and Genes."

Amen, Daniel G. 2017. *Memory Rescue: Supercharge Your Brain, Reverse Memory Loss, and Remember What Matters Most*. Carol Stream, IL: Tyndale Momentum Books.

Appleby, B.S., et al. 2013. "Treatment of Alzheimer's Disease Discovered in Repurposed Agents." *Dementia and Geriatric Cognitive Disorders* 35: 1–22. doi.org/10.1159/000345791.

BAI Beacon. 2017. "The Role of Genetics: Will I Get Alzheimer's Disease?" *End Alzheimer's Now News*, 1 June.

Balin, Brian, et al. 1998. "Identification and Localization of *Chlamydia pneumoniae* in the Alzheimer's Brain." *Medical Microbiology and Immunology* 187: 23–42.

Balin, Brian, et al. 2018. "*Chlamydia pneumoniae*: An Etiologic Agent for Late-Onset Dementia." *Frontiers in Aging Neuroscience* 10, no. 302 (9 October). doi.org/10.3389/fnagi.2018.00302.

Barnes, Lisa, et al. 2015. "Cytomegalovirus Infection and Risk of Alzheimer Disease in Older Black and White Individuals." *Journal of Infectious Diseases* 211, no. 2 (January): 230–37. doi:10.1093/infdis/jiu437.

Begley, Sharon. 2018. "How an Outsider in Alzheimer's Research Bucked the Prevailing Theory—and Clawed for Validation." *STAT*, 29 October. https://www.statnews.com/2018/10/29/alzheimers-research-outsider-bucked-prevailing-theory/.

Begum, Nasrin, et al. 2012. "Does Ionizing Radiation Influence Alzheimer's Disease Risk?" *Journal of Radiation Research* 53, no. 6 (November): 815–22. doi:10.1093/jrr/rrs036.

Bekris, Lynn M., et al. 2010. "Genetics of Alzheimer Disease." *Journal of Geriatric Psychiatry and Neurology* 23, no. 4 (December): 213–27. doi:10.1177/0891988710383571.

Bhandari, Tamara. 2018. "Antibiotic Use Increases Risk of Severe Viral Disease in Mice: Killing Gut Bacteria with Drugs Weakens Immune Response." *Washington University School of Medicine in St. Louis News Release*, 27 March. https://medicine.wustl.edu/news/antibiotic-use-increases-risk-of-severe-viral-disease-in-mice/.

Blagosklonny, Mikhail V. 2017 "From Rapalogs to Anti-Aging Formula." *Oncotarget* 8, no. 22 (30 May): 35492–507. doi:10.18632/oncotarget.18033.

Blennow, Kaj, and Henrik Zetterberg. 2015. "The Past and the Future of Alzheimer's Disease CSF Biomarkers: A Journey toward Validated Biochemical Tests Covering the Whole Spectrum of Molecular Events." *Frontiers in Neuroscience* 9, no. 345 (September): doi:10.3389/fnins.2015.00345.

Bone, Eugenia. 2018. *Microbia: A Journey into the Unseen World around You.* New York: Rodale Books.

Bredesen, Dale. 2017. *The End of Alzheimer's: The First Program to Prevent and Reverse Cognitive Decline.* New York: Avery Books.

Brothers, Holly M., et al. 2018. "The Physiological Roles of Amyloid-β Peptide Hint at New Ways to Treat Alzheimer's Disease." *Frontiers in Aging Neuroscience* 10, no. 118: 1–16. doi:10.3389/fnagi.2018.00118.

Broxmeyer, Lawrence. 2016. *Alzheimer's Disease: How Its Bacterial Cause Was Found and Then Discarded.* CreateSpace Independent Publishing Platform.

Broxmeyer, Lawrence, and George Perry. 2018. "Alzheimer's: Do Anti-Herpetics Reduce the Risk of Dementia and If So, Why?" *Scientia Ricerca* 2, no. 6.

Brun, Paola, et al. 2018. "Herpes Simplex Virus Type 1 Engages Toll Like Receptor 2 to Recruit Macrophages during Infection of Enteric Neurons." *Frontiers in Microbiology* 9, no. 214 (September). doi:10.3389/fmicb.2018.02148.

Bull, Matthew J., and Nigel T. Plummer. 2014. "Part 1: The Human Gut Microbiome in Health and Disease." *Integrative Medicine: A Clinician's Journal* 13, no. 6 (December): 17–22.

Bull, Matthew J., and Nigel T. Plummer. 2015. "Part 2: Treatments for Chronic Gastrointestinal Disease and Gut Dysbiosis." *Integrative Medicine: A Clinician's Journal* 14, no. 1 (February): 25–33.

Bush, Zach. 2019. "Restore Gut Health: The Science behind a Healthy Gut Microbiome." *Neurohacker Collective*, Microbiome Series, Full Episode Transcript, 29 January.

Chapman University. 2018. "Professor Awarded $2.9 Million Federal Research Grant to Study Alzheimer's Disease." *Chapman University Press Release*, 14 November.

Chen, Vincent Chin-Hung, et al. 2018. "Herpes Zoster and Dementia: A Nationwide Population-Based Cohort Study." *Journal of Clinical Psychiatry* 17, no. 1. doi:10.4088/jcp.16m11312.

Chiti, Fabrizio, and Christopher M. Dobson. 2006. "Protein Misfolding, Functional Amyloid, and Human Disease." *Annual Review of Biochemistry* 75 (July): 333–66. doi.org/10.1146/annurev.biochem.75.101304.123901.

Chow, Vivian, et al. 2010. "An Overview of APP Processing Enzymes and Products." *Neuromolecular Medicine* 12, no. 1 (March): 1–12.

Crew, Bec. 2018. "Marijuana Compound Removes Toxic Alzheimer's Protein from the Brain." *ScienceAlert.com*, 26 May. https://www.sciencealert.com/marijuana-compound-thc-removes-toxic-alzheimer-protein-from-brain.

Crews, Leslie, and Eliezer Masliah. 2010. "Molecular Mechanisms of Neurodegeneration in Alzheimer's Disease." *Human Molecular Genetics* 19, no. R1 (15 April): R12–R20. doi:10.1093/hmg/ddq160.

Currais, Anotonio, et al. 2016. "Amyloid Proteotoxicity Initiates an Inflammatory Response Blocked by Cannabinoids." *Nature Partner Journals: Aging and Mechanisms of Disease* 2, issue 16012 (June). doi:10.1038/npjamd.2016.12.

Dach, Jeffrey, et al. 2015. *Cannabinoid Extracts in Medicine.* Jefferson, NC: McFarland.

Daley, Jason. 2018. "Childhood Virus May Have a Role in Alzheimer's Disease." *Smithsonian.com*, 22 June. www.smithsonianmag.com/smart-news/childhood-virus-may-have-role-alzheimers-disease-180969432/.

Damsker, Jesse M., et al. 2010. "Th1 and Th17 Cells Adversaries and Collaborators." *Annals of the New York Academy of Science* 1183 (January): 211–21. doi:10.1111/j.1749-6632.2009.05133.x.

Davies, Gwynivere, et al. 2006. "Prion Diseases and the Gastrointestinal Tract." *Canadian Journal of Gastroenterology* 20, no. 1 (January): 18–24.

Dementia Care Central. 2019. "Using CBD (Cannabidiol) to Treat the Symptoms of Alzheimer's & Other Dementias." *Dementia Care Central*, 26 February. https://www.dementiacarecentral.com/aboutdementia/treating/cbd.

Devoto, Audra, et al. 2019. "Megaphages Infect Prevotella and Variants Are Widespread in Gut Microbiomes." *Nature Microbiology* 4 (28 January): 693–700. doi:10.1038/s41564-018-0338-9.

Dietert, Rodney. 2016. *The Human Superorganism: How the Microbiome Is Revolutionizing the Pursuit of a Healthy Life*. New York: Dutton, imprint of Random Books.

Ding, Yiming, et al. 2018. "A Deep Learning Model to Predict a Diagnosis of Alzheimer Disease by Using ¹8F-FDG PET of the Brain." *Neuroradiology* 290, no. 2 (6 November). doi.org/10.1148/radiol.2018180958.

Di Paola, Gilbert, and Tae-Wan Kim. 2011. "Linking Lipids to Alzheimer's Disease: Cholesterol and Beyond." *Nature Reviews in Neuroscience* 12 (23 June): 284–96.

Dominguez-Bello, Maria, et al. 2010. "Delivery Mode Shapes the Acquisition and Structure of the Initial Microbiota across Multiple Body Habitats in Newborns." *Proceedings of the National Academy of Sciences of the United States of America* 107, no. 26 (29 June): 11971–75. doi:10.1073/pnas.1002601107.

Dominy, Stephen, et al. 2019. "*Porphyromonas gingivalis* in Alzheimer's Disease Brains: Evidence for Disease Causation and Treatment with Small-Molecule Inhibitors." *Science Advances* 5, no. 1 (23 January). doi:10.1126/sciadv.aau3333.

Dragicevic, N., et al. 2010. "Mitochondrial Amyloid-beta Levels Are Associated with the Extent of Mitochondrial Dysfunction in Different Brain Regions and the Degree of Cognitive Impairment in Alzheimer's Transgenic Mice." *Journal of Alzheimer's Disease* 20, Supplement 2: S535-50. doi:10.3233/JAD-2010-100342.

Eccles, John, ed. 1966. *Brain and Conscious Experience: Study Week September 28 to October 4, 1964, of the Pontificia Academia Scientarium*. Berlin: Springer-Verlag.

Eccles, John. 1991. *Evolution of the Brain, Creation of the Self*. London: Routledge.

Eimer, William A., et al. 2018. "Alzheimer's Disease-Associated β-Amyloid Is Rapidly Seeded by *Herpesviridae* to Protect against Brain Infection." *Neuron* 99, no. 1 (11 July): 56–63. doi:10.1016/j.neuron.2018.06.030.

Ellison, James. 2018. "Gut Bacteria and Brains: How the Microbiome Affects Alzheimer's Disease." *Bright Focus Foundation*, 23 March. https://www.brightfocus.org/alzheimers/article/gut-bacteria-and-brains-how-microbiome-affects-alzheimers-disease.

Engelkirk, Paul, and Janet Duben-Engelkirk. 2015. *Burton's Microbiology for the Health Sciences*. 10th ed. Philadelphia: Wolters Kluwer Health, a Division of Lippincot, Williams & Wilkins.

Estep, Preston. 2016. "The Mindspan Diet: The Book Brigade Talks to Geneticist Preston Estep about Eating for Your Brain." *The Book Brigade, Author Speaks*, 27 September.

Ewaleifoh, Osefame, et al. 2017. "TLR3 Elicits Constitutive HSV-1 Resistance in Human Cortical Neurons and Inducible Resistance in Trigeminal Neurons." *Journal of Immunology*, presented at the Madridge's International Conference on Immunology and Immunotechnology. https://madridge.org/journal-of-immunology/immunology-2017-accepted-proceedings/2638-2024.a1.004-a008.pdf.

Farooq, Iqra. 2018. "Why Are BACE Inhibitors Failing Clinical Trials?" *European Pharmaceutical Review*, 31 July. https://www.europeanpharmaceuticalreview.com/news/77751/bace-clinical-trials/.

Fenlon, Wesley. 2013. "The Oligodynamic Effect: How Some Metals Kill Off Bacteria." *Tested*, 7 March.

Fifield, Kathleen. 2019. "New Report Pans Supplements for Brain Health." *AARP Collaborative Council*, 11 June.

Fu, Jingyuan, et al. 2015. "The Gut Microbiome Contributes to a Substantial Proportion of the

Variation in Blood Lipids." *Circulation Research* 117, no. 9 (9 October): 817–24. doi:10.1161/CIRCRESAHA.115.306807.

Fülöp, Támas, et al. 2018. "Can an Infection Hypothesis Explain the Beta Amyloid Hypothesis of Alzheimer's Disease?" *Frontiers in Aging Neuroscience* 10, no. 224 (24 July). www.ncbi.nlm.nih.gov/pmc/articles/PMC6066504/.

Fülöp, Támas, et al. 2018. "Role of Microbes in the Development of Alzheimer's Disease: State of the Art—An International Symposium Presented at the 2017 IAGG Congress in San Francisco." *Frontiers in Genetics* 9, no. 362 (September). doi:10.3389/fgene.2018.00362; www.ncbi.nlm.nih.gov/pmc/articles/PMC6139345/.

Ganz, Tomas. 2013. "The Role of Antimicrobial Peptides in Innate Immunity." *Integrative and Comparative Biology* 43, no. 2 (April): 300–304. doi.org/10.1093/icb/43.2.300.

Ganziga, Michael S. 2018. *The Consciousness Instinct: Unraveling the Mystery of How the Brain Makes the Mind.* New York: Farrar, Strauss.

Gao, Lu, et al. 2018. "Oral Microbiomes: More and More Importance in Oral Cavity and Whole Body." *Protein & Cell* 9, no. 5 (May): 488–500. doi:10.1007/s13238-0180-0548-1.

Geschwind, Michael D., et al. 2007. "Rapidly Progressive Dementia." *Neurologic Clinics* 25, no. 3 (August): 783–803. doi:10.1016/j.ncl.2007.04.001.

Goldfine, Howard. 2018. "Cytochrome *c* Takes on Plasmalogen Catabolism." *Journal of Biological Chemistry* 293, no. 22 (1 June): 8710–11. doi:10.1074/jbc.H118.003072.

Gordon, Jeffrey I., et al. 2006. "Extending Our View of Self: The Human Gut Microbiome Initiative (HGMI)." *Press Release from the Center for Genome Sciences, Washington University* (January). https://www.genome.gov/Pages/Research/Sequencing/SeqProposals/HGMISeq.pdf.

Goschorska, Marta, et al. 2018. "Potential Role of Fluoride in the Etiopathogenesis of Alzheimer's Disease." *International Journal of Molecular Sciences* 19, no. 12 (December). doi:10.3390/ijms19123965.

Gosztyla, Maya L., et al. 2018. "Alzheimer's Amyloid-β Is an Antimicrobial Peptide: A Review of the Evidence." *Journal of Alzheimer's Disease* 62, no. 4 (February): 1495–1506. doi:10.3233/JAD-171133.

Grandjean, Phillipe, and Philip J. Landrigan. 2014. "Neurobehavioral Effects of Developmental Toxicity." *Lancet Neurology* 13 (15 February): 330–38. doi.org/10.1016/S1474-4422(13)70278-3.

Gratuze, Maud, et al. 2018. "New Insights into the Role of TREM2 in Alzheimer's Disease." *Molecular Neurodegeneration* (December). doi.org/10.1186/a13024-018-0298-9.

Gray, Michael W. 2015. "Mosaic Nature of the Mitochondrial Proteome: Implications for the Origin and Evolution of Mitochondria." *Proceedings of the National Academy of Sciences of the United States of America* 112, no. 33 (18 August): 10133–38. doi.org/10.1073/pnas.1421379112.

Green, Alan. 2018. "Introduction to Off-Label Use of Rapamycin / APOE4 Carrier, the Alzheimer's Disease Story." https://alzheimer-prevention.com/.

Guffey, David, et al. 2017. "Herpes Zoster Following Varicella Vaccination in Children." *Cutis* 99, no. 3 (March): 207–11. https://www.mdedge.com/dermatology/article/132772/pediatrics/herpes-zoster-following-varicella-vaccination-children.

Gundry, Steven R. 2019. *The Longevity Paradox: How to Die Young at a Ripe Old Age.* New York: Harper Wave, Imprint of HarperCollins.

Gurven, Michael, et al. 2017. "The Tsimane Health and Life History Project: Integrating Anthropology and Biomedicine." *Evolutionary Anthropology* 26, no. 2 (March–April): 54–73. doi:10.1002/evan.21515.

Haas, Laura, and Stephen Strittmatter. 2016. "Oligomers of Amyloid β Prevent Physiological Activation of the Cellular Prion Protein-Metabotropic Glutamate Receptor 5 Complex by Glutamate in Alzheimer Disease." *Journal of Biological Chemistry* 33 (12 August): 17112–21. doi:10.1074/jbc.M116.720664.

Haas, Laura, et al. 2016. "Metabotropic Glutamate Receptor 5 Couples Cellular Prion Protein to Intracellular Signaling in Alzheimer's Disease." *Brain* 139, no. 2 (February): 526–46. doi:10.1093/brain/awv356.

Haran, J.P., et al. 2019. "Alzheimer's Disease Microbiome Is Associated with Dysregulation of the Anti-Inflammatory P-Glycoprotein Pathway." *MBio American Society of Microbiology* 10, no. 3 (7 May). doi:10.1128/mBio.00632-19.

Harmon, Katherine. 2009. "Bugs Inside: What Happens When the Microbes That Keep Us Healthy Disappear?" *Scientific American*, 16 December.

Harris, Steven, and Elizabeth Harris. 2018. "Molecular Mechanisms for Herpes Simplex Virus Type 1 Pathogenesis in Alzheimer's Disease." *Frontiers in Aging Neuroscience* 10, no. 48 (March). doi:10.3389/fnagi.2018.00048.

Heckman, George A., et al. 2004. "Rapidly Progressive Dementia Due to *Mycobacterium neoaurum* Meningoencephalitis." *Emerging Infectious Diseases* 10, no. 5 (May): 924–27. doi:10.3201/eid1005.030711.

Heine, Steven J. 2017. *DNA Is Not Destiny: The Remarkable, Completely Misunderstood Relationship between You and Your Genes.* New York: Norton.

Hicks, Kristen. 2018. "The Connection between Alzheimer's and Hearing Loss." *Alzheimers. net* (blog), 13 April. https://www.alzheimers.net/the-connection-between-alzheimers-and-hearing-loss/.

Hill, James, and Walter Lukiw. 2015. "Microbial-Generated Amyloids and Alzheimer's Disease." *Frontiers in Aging Neuroscience* (10 February). doi.org/10.3389/fnagi.2015.00009.

Hill, James, et al. 2014. "Pathogenic Microbes, the Microbiome, and Alzheimer's Disease (AD)." *Frontiers in Aging Neuroscience* 6, no. 127 (June): 1–5. doi:10.3389/fnagi.2014.00127.

Hillis, Krista. 2015. "Alzheimer's Statistics—United States & Worldwide Stats." *Brain Test.* https://braintest.com/alzheimers-statistics-throughout-the-united-states-and-worldwide/.

Hirai, Keisuke, et al. 2001. "Mitochondrial Abnormalities in Alzheimer's Disease." *Journal of Neuroscience: The Official Journal of the Society for Neuroscience* 21, no. 9 (June): 3017–23. doi:10.1017/S1431927611001875.

Holmes, C., et al. 2003. "Systemic Infection, Interleukin 1β, and Cognitive Decline in Alzheimer's Disease." *Journal of Neurology, Neurosurgery, and Psychiatry* 74: 788–89.

Hopperton, K. E., et al. 2018. "Markers of Microglia in Post-mortem Brain Samples from Patients with Alzheimer's Disease: A Systematic Review." *Molecular Psychiatry* 23, no. 2 (February): 177–98. doi:10/1038/mp.2017.246.

Hou, Yujun, et al. 2018. "NAD$^+$ Supplementation Normalizes Key Alzheimer's Features and DNA Damage Responses in a New AD Mouse Model with Introduced DNA Repair Deficiency." *Proceedings of the National Academy of Sciences of the United States of America* 115, no. 8 (20 February). doi.org/10.1073/pnas.1718819115, pnas.org/content/115/8/E1876.

Hunt, Tam. 2019. "Interview with Professor Morgan Levine." *Lifespan.Io Interviews*, 18 June. https://www.leafscience.org/interview-with-prof-morgan-levine/.

Hyman, Mark. 2019. "The Problem with Our Vanishing Bacteria." Email from *brokenbrain. com*, 14 June.

Iizuka, Tomomichi, et al. 2017. "Preventive Effect of Rifampicin on Alzheimer Disease Needs at Least 450 mg Daily for 1 Year: An FDG-PET Follow-Up Study." *Dementia and Cognitive Disorders Extra* 7, no. 2 (May–August): 204–14. doi:10.1159/000477343.

Itzhaki, Ruth. 2018. "Corroboration of a Major Role for Herpes Simplex Virus Type 1 in Alzheimer's Disease." *Frontiers in Aging Neuroscience* 10, no. 324. doi:10.3389/fnagi.2018.00324.

Itzhaki, Ruth, and Richard Lathe. 2018. "Herpes Viruses and Senile Dementia: First Population Evidence for a Causal Link." *Journal of Alzheimer's Disease* 64, no. 2: 363–66. doi:10.3233/JAD-180266.

Itzhaki, Ruth, et al. 2016. "Microbes and Alzheimer's Disease." *Journal of Alzheimer's Disease* 51, no. 4 (March): 979–84. doi:10.3233/JAD-160152.

Ivanov, Ivaylo, et al. 2019. "Induction of Intestinal Th17 Cells by Segmented Filamentous Bacteria." *Cell* 139, no. 3 (30 October): 485–98. doi:10.1016/j.cell.2009.09.033.

Jack, Clifford, et al. 2016. "A/T/N: An Unbiased Descriptive Classification Scheme for Alzheimer Disease Biomarkers." *Neurology* 87: 539–57.

Jonsson, Thorlakur, et al. 2012. "A Muation in APP Protects Against Alzheimer's Disease and Age-Related Cognitive Decline." Letter in *Nature* (11 July). doi:10.1038/nature11283.

Kabba, John Alimamy, et al. 2018. "Microglia: Housekeeper of the Central Nervous System." *Cellular and Molecular Neurobiology* 38, no. 1 (January): 53–71. doi.org/10.1007/s10571-017-0504-2.

Kaeberlein, Matt, and Veronica Galvan. 2019. "Rapamycin and Alzheimer's Disease: Time for a Clinical Trial." *Science Translational Medicine* 11, issue 476 (23 January). doi:10.1126/scitranslmed.aar4289.

Kamer, Angela, et al. 2010. "TNF-α and Antibodies to Periodontal Bacteria Discriminate between Alzheimer's Disease Patients and Normal Subjects." *Journal of Neuroimmunology* 216, no. 1–2 (30 November): 92–97. doi:10.1016/j.neuroim.2009.08.013.

Kandel, Eric R. 2018. *The Disordered Mind.* New York: Farrar, Straus, and Giroux.

Kandel, Eric R., et al., eds. 2000. *Principles of Neural Science.* 4th edition. New York: McGraw-Hill.

Kaufmann, Sandra. 2017. *The Kaufmann Protocol: Why We Age and How to Stop It.* Kaufmann Anti-Aging Institute.

Kawahara, Masahiro, and Midori Kato-Negishi, 2011. "Link Between Aluminum and the Pathogenesis of Alzheimer's Disease: The Integration of the Aluminum and Amyloid Cascade Hypotheses." *International Journal of Alzheimer's Disease* (March). doi:10.4061/2011/276393.

Keele University. 2014. "Elevated Brain Aluminum, Early Onset Alzheimer's Disease in an Individual Occupationally Exposed to Aluminum." *Science Daily*, 12 February.

Khan, Mohsin, et al. 2015. "Mitochondrial Dynamics and Viral Infections: A Close Nexus." *Biochimica et Biophysica Acta (BBA)—Molecular Cell Research*, Part B, 1853, no. 10 (October): 2822–33. doi.org/10.1016/j.bbamcr.2014.12.040.

Kowalski, Karol, and Agata Mulak. 2019. "Brain-Gut-Microbiota Axis in Alzheimer's Disease." *Journal of Neurogastroenterology and Motility* 25, no. 1 (January): 48–60.

Kristoferitsch, Wolfgang, et al. 2018. "Secondary Dementia Due to Lyme Neuroborreliosis." *Wiener klinische Wochenschrift (The Central European Journal of Medicine)* 130, no. 15: 468–78. doi.1007/s00508-018-1361-9.

Kumar, Anil, and Nikita Chordia. 2017. "Role of Microbes in Human Health." *Applied Microbiology: Open Access* 3, no. 1: 1–5. doi:10.4172/2471-9315.1000131.

Lam, A.D., et al. 2017. "Silent Hippocampal Seizures and Spikes Identified by Foramen Ovale Electrodes in Alzheimer's Disease." *Nature Medicine* 23, no. 6 (June): 678–80. doi:10.1038/nm.4330.

Langelier, Julie. 2018. "Scientists Find a New Way to Attack Herpesviruses." *Medical Xpress*, 28 August. https://medicalxpress.com/news/2018-08-scientists-herpesviruses.html.

LaRosa, Francesca, et al. 2018. "The Gut-Brain Axis in Alzheimer's Disease and Omega-3: A Critical Overview of Clinical Trials." *Nutrients* 10, no. 1267 (8 September): 1–17. doi:10.3390/nu10091267.

Leheste, Joerg, et al. 2017. "*P. acnes*–Driven Disease Pathology: Current Knowledge and Future Directions." *Frontiers in Cell Infection and Microbiology* 7, no. 81 (14 March). doi:10.3389/fcimb.2017.00081.

Levine, Morgan E., et al. 2018. "An Epigenetic Biomarker of Aging for Lifespan and Healthspan." *Aging* 10, no. 4 (April): 573–91. doi:10.18632/aging.101414.

Life Extension Staff. 2018. "Protect Your Memory & Stay Sharp." *Life Extension Health Digest: The Science of Great Health* (December): 8–9.

Lioret, Ana, et al. 2019. "The Effectiveness of Vitamin E Treatment in Alzheimer's Disease." *International Journal of Molecular Science* 20, no. 4 (February). doi:10.3390/ifms2004879.

Livingston, Gill, et al. 2017. "The Lancet International Commission on Dementia Prevention and Care." *Lancet* 16, no. 390 (December): 2673–74.

Lövheim, H., et al. 2018. "Interaction between Cytomegalovirus and Herpes Simplex Virus Type 1 Associated with the Risk of Alzheimer's Disease Development." *Journal of Alzheimer's Disease* 68, no. 3: 939–45. doi:10.3233/JAD-161305.

Lozupone, Catherine, et al. 2012. "Diversity, Stability, and Resilience of the Human Gut Microbiota." *Nature* 489, no. 7415 (13 September): 220–30. doi:10.1038/nature11550.

Lurain, Nell, et al. 2013. "Virological and Immunological Characteristics of Human Cytomegalovirus Infection Associated with Alzheimer Disease." *Journal of Infectious Diseases* 208, no. 4 (August): 564–72. doi.org/10.1093/infdis/jit210.

Ma, F., et al. 2017. "Effects of Folic Acid Supplementation on Cognitive Function and Aβ-Related Biomarkers in Mild Cognitive Impairment: A Randomized Controlled Trial." *European Journal of Nutrition.*

MacDonald, Alan. 2016. "Alzheimer's Disease Brain Contains Nematode Parasites with *Endosymbiont Borrelia* Microbes Inside of Worm Parasites Part One: Trichrome Stains of Worms in Alzheimer Hippocampus." *F1000Research: Open for Science*, 14 June. doi. org/10.7490/f1000research.1112323.1.

Markel, Howard. 2004. *When Germs Travel: Major Epidemics That Have Invaded America Since 1900 and the Fears They Have Unleashed.* New York: Pantheon Books.

Matsuyama, Kanoko. 2019. "A Blood Test Can Predict Dementia. Trouble Is, There's No Cure." *Bloomberg.com*, 21 May. https://www.bloomberg.com/news/articles/2019-05-21/a-blood-test-can-predict-dementia-trouble-is-there-s-no-cure.

Mawanda, Francis, and Robert Wallace. 2013. "Can Infections Cause Alzheimer's Disease?" *Epidemiologic Reviews* 35, no. 1 (January): 161–80. doi:10.1093/epirev/mxs007.

McKeehan, Nick. 2019. "Sleep and Alzheimer's Disease: More Evidence on Their Relationship." *Alzheimer's Drug Discovery Foundation*, 6 February. https://www.alzdiscovery. org/cognitive-vitality/blog/sleep-and-alzheimers-disease-more-evidence-on-their-relationship.

McManus, Roisin M., and Michael T. Heneka. 2017. "Role of Neuroinflammation in Neurodegeneration: New Insights." *Alzheimer's Research & Therapy* 9, no. 14 (4 March). doi. org/10.1186/s13195-017-0241-2.

Mercier-Darty, M., et al. 2018. "Utility of Ultra-deep Sequencing for Detection of Varicella-Zoster Virus Antiviral Resistance Mutations." *Antiviral Resistance* 151 (March): 20–23. doi:10.1016/j.antiviral.2018.01.008.

Miklossy, Judith. 2017. "Alzheimer's Disease and Spirochetosis: A Causal Relationship." *Journal of Alzheimer's Disease* (27 February).

Miller, Alan. 2018. "What Is Methylation and Why Should You Care About It." *Thorne Take 5 Daily*, 3 September.

Miller, F., et al. 2012. "Blood-Brain Barrier and Retroviral Infections." *Virulence* 3, no. 2 (1 March): 222–29. doi:10.4161/viru.19697, https://www.ncbi.nlm.nih.gov/pmc/articles/PMC3396701/.

Mitteldorf, Josh. 2019. "DNAm GrimAge; The Newest Methylation Clock; Methylation Update Part II." *Aging Matters* (5 March).

Moir, Robert, et al. 2018. "The Antimicrobial Protection Hypothesis of Alzheimer's Disease." *Alzheimer's & Dementia: The Journal of the Alzheimer's Association* 14, no. 12: 1602–14. doi:https://doi.org/10.1016/j.jalz.2018.06.3040.

Monsonego, Alon, et al. 2013. "CD4+ T Cells in Immunity and Immunotherapy of Alzheimer's Disease." *Immunology* 139, no. 4 (August): 438–46. doi:10.1111/imm.12103.

Morgan, Paul. 2017. "Complement in the Pathogenesis of Alzheimer's Disease." *Seminars in Immunopathology* 40, no. 1 (13 November): 113–24. doi:10.1007/s00281-017-0662-9.

Morimoto, Kaori, et al. 2013. "Expression Profiles of Cytokines in the Brains of Alzheimer's Disease (AD) Patients, Compared to the Brains of Non-demented Patients with and Without Increasing AD Pathology." *Journal of Alzheimer's Disease* 25, no. 1 (14 February): 59–76. doi:10.3233/JAD-2011-101815.

Mushegian, Sasha. 2018. "What Happens to Plasmalogens, the Phospholipids Nobody Likes to Think About." *Journal of Biological Chemistry* (1 November).

Mutter, J., et al. 2010. "Does Inorganic Mercury Play a Role in Alzheimer's Disease? A Systematic Review and an Integrated Molecular Mechanism." *Journal of Alzheimer's Disease* 22, no. 2: 357–74. doi:10.3233/JAD-2010-100705.

Myslinski, Norbert. 2014. "Alzheimer's Disease and the Blood-Brain Barrier." *Today's Geriatric Medicine* 7, no. 1 (January–February). http://www.todaysgeriatricmedicine.com/archive/012014p26.shtml.

Natawala, A., et al. 2008. "Reasons for Hospital Admissions in Dementia Patients in Birmingham, UK, during 2002–2007." *Dementia and Geriatric Cognitive Disorders* 26: 499–505. doi:10.1159/000171044.

Nation, Daniel, et al. 2019. "Blood-Brain Barrier Breakdown Is an Early Biomarker of Human Cognitive Dysfunction." *Nature Medicine* 25 (January): 270–76. doi.org/10.1038/s41591-018-0297-y.

Ngo, Huan, et al. 2017. "*Toxoplasma* Modulates Signature Pathways of Human Epilepsy,

Neurodegeneration & Cancer." *Scientific Reports* 7, no. 1 (13 September). doi:10.1038 /s41598-017-10675-6.

Nicolson, Garth. 2014. "Mitochondrial Dysfunction and Chronic Disease: Treatment with Natural Supplements." *Integrative Medicine: A Clinician's Journal* 12, no. 4 (August): 35–43.

Nobel Prize Awards. www.nobelprize.org/prizes/lists/all-nobel-prizes/.

Nwanaji-Enwerem, Jamaji C., et al. 2016. "Long-term Ambient Particle Exposures and Blood DNA Methylation Age: Findings from the VA Normative Aging Study." *Environmental Epigenetics* 2, no. 2 (April). doi:10.1093/eep/dvw006.

Oberstein, Timo Jan, et al. 2018. "Imbalance of Circulating $T_h17$ and Regulatory T Cells in Alzheimer's Disease: A Case Control Study." *Frontiers in Immunology* (4 June). doi. org/10.3389/fimmu.2018.01213.

Parady, Bodo. 2018. "Innate Immune and Fungal Model of Alzheimer's Disease." *Journal of Alzheimer's Disease Reports* 2, no. 1 (26 July): 139–52. doi:10.3233/ADR-180073.

Parthasarathy, Geetha, and Mario T. Phillipp. 2012. "Apoptotic Mechanisms in Bacterial Infections of the Central Nervous System." *Frontiers in Immunology* (4 October). doi:10.3389/ fimmu.2012.00306.

Penfield, W., and B. Milner. 1958. "Memory Deficit Produced by Bilateral Lesions in the Hippocampal Zone." *American Medical Association Archives of Neurology and Psychiatry* 79, no. 5 (May): 475–97.

Perlmutter, David. 2013. *Grain Brain.* New York: Little, Brown.

Piacentini, Roberto, et al. 2014. "HSV-1 and Alzheimer's Disease: More Than a Hypothesis." *Frontiers in Pharmacology* 5, no. 97 (May). doi:10.3389/fphar.2014.00097.

Pirker-Kees, Agnes, et al. 2013. "T-Cells Show Increased Production of Cytokines and Activation Markers in Alzheimer's Disease." *Brain Disorders and Therapy* 3, no. 112 (20 December). doi:10.4172/2168-975X.1000112.

Pisa, Diana, et al. 2015. "Different Brain Regions Are Infected with Fungi in Alzheimer's Disease." *Scientific Reports* 5, no. 15015. doi:10.1038/srep15015.

Powell, Alvin. 2017. "Probe of Alzheimer's Follows Paths of Infection: Starting with Microbes, Harvard-MGH Researchers Outline a Devastating Chain of Events." *Harvard Gazette,* 11 May.

Pretorius, Etheresia, et al. 2016. "A Bacterial Component to Alzheimer's-Type Dementia Seen with a Systems Biology Approach That Links Iron Dysregulation and Inflammagen Shedding to Disease." *Journal of Alzheimer's Disease* 53, no. 4: 1237–56. doi:10.3233/JAD-160318.

Proal, Amy. 2017. "Interview with Robert Moir: Infection in Alzheimer's/Brain Microbiome." *Microbe Minded* (18 December).

Qin, Junjie. 2010. "A Human Gut Microbial Gene Catalogue Established by Metagenomic Sequencing." *Nature* 464 (4 March): 59–65.

Quetel, Claude. 1990. *History of Syphilis.* Translated by Judith Braddock and Brian Pike. First published in France as *Le Mal de Naples; histoire de la syphilis* (Editions Seghers, 1986). Baltimore: Johns Hopkins University Press, 1990.

Rak, K., et al. 2014. "Neurotrophic Effects of Taurine on Spiral Ganglion Neurons in Vitro." *Neuroreport* 25, no. 16 (November): 1250–54.

Ramos-Cejudo, J., et al. 2018. "Traumatic Brain Injury and Alzheimer's Disease: The Cerebrovascular Link." *EBiomedicine* 28 (February): 21–30. doi:10.1016/j.ebiom.2018.01.021.

Redd, Nola. 2019. "How Old Is Earth?" *Space.com,* 7 February. www.space.com/24854-how-old-is-earth.html.

Rose, Hilary, and Steven Rose. 2012. *Genes, Cells and Brains: The Promethean Promises of the New Biology.* London: Verso.

Rybakowski, Janusz K. 2019. "Commentary: Corroboration of a Major Role for Herpes Simplex Virus Type 1 in Alzheimer's Disease." *Frontiers in Aging Neuroscience* 10, no. 433 (10 January). doi:10.3380/fnagi.2018.00433.

Salvaggio, Michelle. 2018. "Human Herpesvirus 6 (HHV-6) Infection." *Medscape,* 29 November. https://emedicine.medscape.com/article/219019-overview.

Sanders, Robert, et al. 2008. "Biologic Effects of Nitrous Oxide: A Mechanistic and Toxicologic Review." *Anesthesiology* 109 (October): 707–22. doi:10.1097/ALN.0b013e3181870a17.

Santos, Renato, et al. 2013. "Mitochondrial DNA Oxidative Damage and Repair in Aging and Alzheimer's Disease." *Antioxidants & Redox Signaling* 18, no. 8 (20 June): 2244–57. doi:10.1089/ars.2012.5039.

Satizibal, C. L., et al. 2016. "Incidence of Dementia Over Three Decades in the Framingham Heart Study." *New England Journal of Medicine* 374, no. 6 (11 February): 523–32. doi:10.1056/NEJMoa1504327.

Sauer, Alissa. 2017. "Has Alzheimer's Always Impacted Humanity? A Look at an Ancient Cure." *Alzheimers.net* (blog), 27 September. https://www.alzheimers.net/alzheimers-impacted-humanity/.

Scarpellini, Emidio, et al. 2015. "The Human Gut Microbiota and Virome: Potential Therapeutic Implications." *Liver and Digestive Diseases* 47, no. 12 (December): 1007–12. doi:https://doi.org/10.1016/j.dld.2015.07.008.

Sellami, Maha, et al. 2018. "Effects of Acute and Chronic Exercise on Immunological Parameters in the Elderly Aged: Can Physical Activity Counteract the Effects of Aging?" *Frontiers in Immunology* 9, no. 2187 (10 October). doi.org/10.3389/fimmu.2018.02187.

Serino, M., et al. 2012. "Microbes On-Air Gut and Tissue Microbiota as Targets in Type 2 Diabetes." *Journal of Clinical Gastroenterology* 46, no. 9 (October), Supplement: S27–S28.

Seshadri, Sudha, et al. 2002. "Plasma Homocysteine as a Risk Factor for Dementia and Alzheimer's Disease." *New England Journal of Medicine* 346, no. 7 (14 February): 476–83. doi:10.1056/NEJMoa011613.

Shahar, S., et al. 2013. "Association Between Vitamin A, Vitamin E and Apolipoprotein E Status with Mild Cognitive Impairment Among Elderly People in Low-Cost Residential Areas." *Nutritional Neuroscience* 16, no. 1 (January). doi:10.1179/1476830512Y.0000000013.

Shal, Bushra, et al. 2018. "Anti-neuroinflammatory Potential of Natural Products in Attenuation of Alzheimer's Disease." *Frontiers in Pharmacology* (29 May). doi.org/10.3389/fphar.2018.00548.

Sherzai, Dean, and Ayesha Sherzai. 2017. *The Alzheimer's Solution: A Breakthrough Program to Prevent and Reverse the Symptoms of Cognitive Decline at Every Age.* New York: HarperCollins.

Shi, Liu, et al. 2018. "A Decade of Blood Biomarkers for Alzheimer's Disease Research: An Evolving Field, Improving Study Designs, and the Challenge of Replication." *Journal of Alzheimer's Disease* 62, no. 3 (13 March): 1181–98. doi:10.3233/JAD-170531.

Shim, Sung-Mi, et al. 2017. "Elevated Epstein-Barr Virus Antibody Level Is Associated with Cognitive Decline in the Korean Elderly." *Journal of Alzheimer's Disease* 55, no. 1: 293–301.

Shoemark, Deborah, and Shelley J. Allen. 2015. "The Microbiome and Disease: Reviewing the Links Between the Oral Microbiome, Aging, and Alzheimer's Disease." *Journal of Alzheimer's Disease* 43: 725–38. doi:10.323/JAD-141170.

Smith, Patrick M., et al. 2013. "The Microbial Metabolites, Short Chain Fatty Acids, Regulate Colonic Treg Cell Homeostasis." *Science* 341, no. 6145 (4 July). doi:10.1126/science.1241165.

Sochocka, Marta, et al. 2017. "The Infectious Etiology of Alzheimer's Disease." *Current Neuropharmacology* 15, no. 7 (October): 996–1009. doi:10.2174/1570159X15666170313122937.

Sochocka, Marta, et al. 2018. "The Gut Microbiome Alterations and Inflammation-Driven Pathogenesis of Alzheimer's Disease: A Critical Review." *Molecular Neurobiology* (23 June): 1–11. doi.org/10.1007/s12035-018-1188-4.

Srisruknimit, Veerasak. 2018. "Fighting Fire with Fire: Killing Bacteria with Viruses." *Harvard University Science in the News* (blog), 1 February. http://sitn.hms.harvard.edu/flash/2018/bacteriophage-solution-antibiotics-problem/.

Stamouli, E.C., and A.M. Politis. 2016. "Pro-inflammatory Cytokines in Alzheimer's Disease." *Psychiatriki* 27, no. 4 (October–December): 264–75. doi:10.22365/jpsych.2016.274.264.

Stetka, Bret S. 2018. "Infectious Theory of Alzheimer Disease Draws Fresh Interest." *Medscape Neurology* (14 November).

Strait, Julia Evangelou, 2017. "The Father of the Microbiome." *The Source* (Washington University in S. Louis), 3 March. https://source.wustl.edu/2017/03/the-father-of-the-microbiome/.

Stromrud, Erik, et al. 2010. "Alterations of Matrix Metalloproteinases in the Healthy Elderly with Increased Risk of Prodromal Alzheimer's Disease." *Alzheimer's Research & Therapy* 2, no. 20: doi:10.1186/alzrt44.

Swaab, D. F. 2014. *We Are Our Brains: A Neurobiography of the Brain from the Womb to Alzheimer's*. Translated by Jane Hedley-Prôle. New York: Spiegel and Grau.

Sweeney, Melanie D., et al. 2018. "Blood-Brain Barrier Breakdown in Alzheimer Disease and Other Neurodegenerative Disorders." *Nature Reviews in Neurology* 14 (January): 133–50.

Swerdlow, Russell H. 2018. "Mitochondria and Mitochondrial Cascades in Alzheimer's Disease." *Journal of Alzheimer's Disease* 62, no. 3 (13 March): 1403–16. doi:10.3233/JAD-170585.

Tanzi, Rudolph E., and Lars Bertram. 2001. "New Frontiers in Alzheimer's Disease Genetics." *Neuron* 32, no. 2 (25 October): 181–84. doi.org/10.1016/S0896-6273(01)00476-7.

Terry, Mark. 2019. "A Blood Test That Can ID Alzheimer's Risk Up to 16 Years Before Symptoms." *Biospace*, 22 January. www.biospace.com/article/possible-predictive-protein-for-alzheimer-s-disease-identified/.

Tetz, George, and Victor Tetz. 2017. "Prion-like Domains in Phagobiota." *Frontiers in Microbiology* 8 (15 November). doi.org/10.3389/fmicb.2017.02239.

Tetz, George, and Victor Tetz. 2018. "Bacteriophages as New Human Viral Pathogens." *Microorganisms* 6, no. 2 (June). doi:10.3390/microorganisms6020054.

Tetzeli, Rick. 2019. "Could This Radical New Approach to Alzheimer's Lead to a Breakthrough?" *Yahoo Finance*, 18 January. https://finance.yahoo.com/news/could-radical-approach-alzheimer-lead-113033328.html.

Thambisetty, Madhav, et al. 2010. "Association of Plasma Clusterin Concentration with Severity, Pathology, and Progression in Alzheimer Disease." *Archives of General Psychiatry* 67, no. 7: 739–48. doi:10.1001/archgenpsychiatry.2010.78.

Townsend, David, et al. 2018. "Epigallocatechin-3-gallate Remodels Apolipoprotein A-I Amyloid Fibrils into Soluble Oligomers in the Presence of Heparin." *Journal of Biological Chemistry* 17, no. 293 (17 August): 12877–93.

Tsai, Ming-Chieh, et al. 2017. "Increased Risk of Dementia Following Herpes Zoster Ophthalmicus." *PLoS One* 12, no. 11 (November). doi:10.1371/journal.pone.0188490.

Tzeng, Nian-Sheng, et al. 2017. "Fibromyalgia and Risk of Dementia—A Nationwide, Population-Based, Cohort Study." *American Journal of the Medical Sciences*. doi:10.1016/j.amjms.2017.09.002.

Uddin, Sahab, et al. 2018. "Autophagy and Alzheimer's Disease: From Molecular Mechanisms to Therapeutic Implications." *Frontiers in Aging Neuroscience* 10, no. 4 (30 January). doi:10.3389/fnagi.2018.00004.

University of California, Davis (UC Davis). 2009. "Alzheimer's Causing Amyloid and Bacteria Trigger Same Immune Response." *UC Davis Health Press Release*, 9 September.

Ursell, Luke K. 2012. "Defining the Human Microbiome." *Nutrition Reviews* 70, Supplement 1 (August): S38–S44.

Vaiserman, Alexander. 2018. "Developmental Tuning of Epigenetic Clock." *Frontiers in Genetics* 22 (November). doi.org/10.3389/fgene.2018.00584.

Vogt, Nicholas, et al. 2017. "Gut Microbiome Alterations in Alzheimer's Disease." *Scientific Reports* 7, no. 13537 (19 October).

Vradenburg, George. 2019. Email from *Us Against Alzheimer's*, 11 June.

Wanucha, Genevieve. 2018. "The Gut Microbiome and Brain Health." *University of Washington Memory and Brain Wellness Center*, 4 October: 1–6. http://depts.washington.edu/mbwc/news/article/the-gut-microbiome-and-brain-health.

Waugh, Declan. 2018. "The Link Between Fluoride Levels and Alzheimer's Disease." *Irish Medical Times*, Letter to the Editor, 22 February.

Weintraub, Karen. 2019. "For Alzheimer's Sufferers, Brain Inflammation Ignites a Neuron-Killing 'Forest Fire': And It Could Also Be the Kindling Sparking Parkinson's and Other Neurodegenerative Maladies." *Scientific American*, 4 March. www.scientificamerican.com/article/for-alzheimers-sufferers-brain-inflammation-ignites-a-neuron-killing-forest-fire/.

Wellcome Trust Sanger Institute. 2019. "More Than 100 New Gut Bacteria Discovered in Human Microbiome: Study Will Help Understand Role of Microbiome in Health and Disease." *Science Daily*, 4 February. www.sciencedaily.com/releases/2019/02/190204114602.htm.

Weyand, Cornelia M., and Jorg J. Goronzy. 2016. "Aging of the Immune System Mechanisms and Therapeutic Targets." *Annals of the American Thoracic Society*, Supplement Transatlantic Airway Conference Publication, Vol. 13, Supplement 5 (December): S422–28. doi:10.1513/AnnalsATS.201602-095AW.

Williams, Anna. 2018. "Human Stem Cell Model Reveals Mechanisms of Herpes Infection." *Northwestern University Medicine: Feinberg School of Medicine News*, 1 October.

World Health Organization. 2019. "Global Tuberculosis Report 2018." https://www.who.int/tb/publications/global_report/en/.

Xu, Shangcheng, et al. 2009. "Exposure to 1800 MHz Radiofrequency Radiation Induces Oxidative Damage to Mitochondrial DNA in Primary Cultured Neurons." *Science Direct* (30 October): 189–96.

Yang, Eun Ju, et al. 2007. "A Clinical Trial of Orally Administered Alkaline Reduced Water." *Journal of Experimental Biomedical Science* 13: 83–89.

Yoo, Brian B., and Sarkis K. Mazmanian. 2017. "The Enteric Network: Interactions Between the Immune and Nervous Systems of the Gut." *Immunity* 46 (20 June): 910–26. doi:https://doi.org/10.1016/j.immuni.2017.05.011.

Zhan, Xinhua, et al. 2018. "Lipopolysaccharide Associates with Amyloid Plaques, Neurons and Oligodendrocytes in Alzheimer's Disease Brain: A Review." *Frontiers in Aging Neuroscience* 10, no. 42 (22 February). doi:10.3389/fnagi.2018.00042.

Zheng, Cong, et al. 2016. "The Dual Roles of Cytokines in Alzheimer's Disease: Update on Interleukins, TNF-α, TGF-β and IFN-γ." *Translations in Neurodegeneration* 5, no. 7 (5 April). doi:10.1186/s40035-016-0054-4.

Zlokovic, Berislav V. 2008. "The Blood-Brain Barrier in Health and Chronic Neurodegenerative Disorders." *Neuron* 1, no. 3. doi:10.1016/j.neuron.2008.01.03.

# Index

Numbers in *bold italics* indicate pages with illustrations

215